Representations of Death

An extraordinary world where the dead are examined, certified, registered, embalmed, viewed and finally cremated or buried is revealed in this ethnographic account of contemporary British mortuary practices. Going behind the scenes, the author explores the interplay between rituals and representations and, in the process, critiques traditional models of grief.

Representations of Death makes use of the social psychological theory of social representations and draws upon fascinating and often poignant data. Illuminating the perspectives of both the grieving relatives and the deathwork professionals, Bradbury shows how talk about a person's death focuses upon its perceived 'goodness' or 'naturalness'. Arguing that these social representations are an expression of our need to make death familiar, she demonstrates how they are anchored and objectified in current mortuary practices.

Illustrated with stunning photographs, *Representations of Death* will be essential reading for anyone interested in death, grief and bereavement.

Mary Bradbury is a researcher and freelance lecturer. She is currently training at the Institute of Psycho-analysis, London.

Representations of Death

A social psychological perspective

Mary Bradbury

Foreword by Robert Farr
Photographs by Peter Rauter

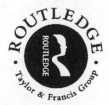

London and New York

First published 1999 by Routledge
2 Park Square, Milton Park, Abingdon, Oxon, OX14 4RN

Simultaneously published in the USA and Canada
by Routledge
711 Third Avenue, New York, NY 10017

Routledge is an imprint of the Taylor & Francis Group

© 1999 Mary Bradbury

Typeset in Garamond by J&L Composition Ltd, Filey,
North Yorkshire

British Library Cataloguing in Publication Data
A catalogue record for this book is available from the British Library

Library of Congress Cataloging in Publication Data

Bradbury, Mary, 1964–
    Representations of death: a social psychological perspective/
Mary Bradbury: foreword by Robert Farr.
        p.   cm
    Includes bibliographical references and index.
    1. Death.   2. Undertakers and undertaking.   3. Funeral
rites and ceremonies.   4. Bereavement.   I. Title.
    HQ1073.B7   1999   99–31070
    306.9—dc21   CIP

ISBN 0-415-15021-3 (hbk)
ISBN 0-415-15022-1 (pbk)

To my parents

Contents

Contents

List of photographs
(before Chapter 5)

Photographs by Peter Rauter

Foreword

Mary Bradbury is a graduate in anthropology of the University of Cambridge and in social psychology of the London School of Economics and Political Science. This, her first book, is based on the fieldwork she undertook in the course of her doctoral studies at the School. Dr Bradbury writes in a highly lucid fashion and her text is refreshingly free of jargon, despite the wealth of scholarship on which it draws. This should make it easily accessible to a wide range of readers such as the professional social scientist, through the complete gamut of health care and deathwork professionals, to lay men and women who, perhaps suddenly, find themselves faced with arranging a funeral. It is also a beautifully illustrated book which deserves to grace the coffee tables of the bourgeoisie (it is, after all, an urban ethnography). The taboo nature of the topic, however, may preclude the appearance of the book actually on the coffee table though, hopefully, it will be ready at hand in a nearby bookcase.

A participant observational study

The illustrations are important for another reason – apart, that is, from making it an attractive volume to purchase. They reflect the participant observational nature of the original study. Dr Bradbury made her observations at some seven different sites associated with the work of various deathwork professionals: funeral parlours, cemeteries, crematoria, intensive care units, registrar's offices, coroner's courts and the headquarters of a murder investigation. These are all spaces within the public sphere. Funerals, *par excellence*, are public events. Goffman (1961), in his essay on some vicissitudes in the history of the tinkering professions, first drew the attention of social scientists to the importance of distinguishing between front and back regions in the social psychology of total institutions. In dealing with death and our mortuary practices in relation to death the separation between front and back of shop is, perhaps, even sharper than in Goffman's model of the doctor–patient relationship.

Going behind the scenes in hospitals (to the morgue, for example), funeral parlours or crematoria is something seldom done by members of the general public (except, perhaps, vicariously in the case of television dramas and then, usually, only in relation to the first of these three sites). Dr Bradbury's account is based on her visits to these sites, together with her conversations with a sample of widows who had recently been bereaved. Her readers gain privileged access to these forbidden regions through the series of black and white photographs illustrating the volume. Some of the photographs may shock some readers, reflecting taboos against making public that which some consider should remain private and beyond the gaze of the public.

It is extremely rare for a study in social psychology to be based on participant observation. The number of such studies, at least in psychological forms of social psychology, can be counted on the fingers of one hand. For significant periods in the history of modern social psychology, the preferred method of research has been the laboratory experiment. Here the social psychologist considers him- or herself to be an observer (in the tradition of a natural scientist) rather than a participant observer. It should scarcely be surprising, then, if most of the artefacts which arise from adopting such a research attitude should be social in nature (Farr 1978).

Social psychologists, like Bradbury, with a professional training in anthropology or sociology, are unlikely to commit such errors. Dr Bradbury remains sensitive throughout to the social psychology of the research process. She is a sympathetic listener, as in her interviews with the recently bereaved, and an astute observer of others, as in her study of deathwork professionals. She is both a participant and an observer in both contexts and knows how to combine these two contrasting perspectives.

The present study is comparable to Jodelet's classic study of madness and its social representations at Aisney-le-Château (Jodelet 1991). Jodelet, too, used participant observation, including fieldnotes, to uncover the representations of madness which lay buried in the customs and rituals of villagers in the region as they accommodated to the mentally ill who had been dwelling among them for some ninety years. Bradbury uses the same theory that Jodelet found useful in explaining her findings, i.e. Moscovici's theory of social representations. Like Jodelet she also relies on being able to interrogate key informants on what it is that she herself has observed to happen. The strength of participant observation as a method of research is that one is not totally dependent on accepting what others may tell one.

The social psychology of a 'rite de passage': death

An important source of inspiration for Bradbury were the studies conducted by Glaser and Strauss on *Awareness of Dying* (1965) and *A Time for Dying* (1968). These were participant observational studies of dying in the context of a cancer ward. These studies were conducted within a sociological form of social psychology, i.e. they were linked to grounded theory and to the symbolic interactionist tradition of social psychology at Chicago. In sociological forms of social psychology participant observation is the norm rather than the exception.

Glaser and Strauss conducted their studies at a time in America when it was becoming increasingly common for patients suffering from cancer to die in hospital rather than at home. The medical staff of a hospital are dedicated to the preservation of life rather than to assisting people to die. The issue of palliative medicine is a later development which is dealt with here by Bradbury in Chapter 3. Glaser and Strauss demonstrate how the strain of nursing the dying patient is borne by the nursing staff of the hospital rather than by medical doctors. While nurses are used to dealing with death in general, for the individual patient who is dying and his/her immediate family death is a unique experience. When a patient dies on the ward the responsibilities of the nursing staff to that particular patient come to an end. Many ward sisters regard it as part of their obligations to their former patient to accompany the corpse to the door of the ward from whence it is then taken to the morgue. This is the point at which they see their responsibilities ceasing. In many respects the present study takes over where the previous study ended, i.e. Mary Bradbury, in her study, then follows the corpse from the time it leaves the ward to the time, about a week later, when it is buried or cremated. This book is an account of that week.

The present volume is an original contribution to Moscovici's theory of social representations. Bradbury sets out the social psychology of an important *rite de passage*, namely, death. Her ethnography is rooted in the Durkheimian tradition. As Bradbury reminds us the objects of study in Wundt's *Völkerpsychologie* (1900–20) were language, religion, customs, ritual, myth, magic and cognate phenomena. These collective mental phenomena are comparable to the collective representations which Durkheim (1898) claimed were the objects of study in sociology. The study of customs, ceremonies and rituals also appeared within the context of the first *Handbook of Social Psychology* edited by Murchison and published in America in 1935. The cultural dimension then rapidly dropped out of the frame, at least in psychological forms of social psychology. Custom became habit and the collective dimension disappeared altogether. Serious scientific research came to focus on the behaviour of white rats and fan-tailed pigeons and culture is fairly minimal at this level of the evolutionary scale.

An anthropology of modern everyday life

When Moscovici resurrected Durkheim's notion of the collective representations at the start of the modern era in social psychology he preferred, for a variety of good reasons, to refer to them as social rather than as collective representations (*Culture and Psychology*, special issue, 1998). He felt that collective representations were more appropriate to an understanding of premodern societies. Social representations, he could claim with some justification, constituted an anthropology of modern everyday life.

In the study of rituals and ceremonies, however, it may still be more appropriate to refer to collective, rather than to social, representations. This is because the ceremonies themselves are collective phenomena. In our ceremonies and rituals we perpetuate the collective representations of yesteryear. Often we are no longer aware of why we do what we do. The structure of the academic year at many UK universities, for example, reflects the fact that members of the faculty need to be back in their parishes for the celebrations of Christmas and Easter and their students need to be back on the land over the summer months to ensure a good harvest. In modernizing Durkheim's notion of collective representations, Moscovici may have made it more difficult to reincorporate the notion of culture within his theory of social representations. The present study is an original contribution to this current debate.

A significant strength of Moscovici's theory of social representations is that it takes seriously both culture and history. These are the forms that space and time assume in the human and social sciences. Mary Bradbury, in this book, traces both the continuities and the discontinuities in British mortuary practices in recent centuries. The most significant change, in her opinion, came with the commercialization of the funeral during the Victorian era and the emergence of the funeral director as Master of Ceremonies at most modern funerals. This fascinating piece of recent social history is the topic of interest in Chapter 4. The laying out of the body in preparation for burial which, previously, was carried out by women in the context of the family home was now handed over to a deathwork professional. During the Victorian era funerals became an occasion for the display of wealth. Bradbury traces some vicissitudes in the history of the deathwork professionals in much the same way as Goffman did for the tinkering professionals. She also has some interesting observations to make on the development of the hospice movement and the growth of pallia-tive, as distinct from remedial, medicine. Her espousal of Moscovici's theory of social representations lends credence to his claim that it is an anthropology of modern life.

Social representations of a good and a bad death

Bloch and Parry (1982), two anthropologists at the London School of Economics, describe the twin notions of a good and a bad death. They speculate that the notions which they analyse in various non-industrial cultures would be meaningless in the context of a highly individu-alized Western metropolis. Bradbury, in her London ethnography, shows that this is not so. Indeed the irony of the situation is that, with the miracles of modern technology, the time and place of death is more or less under medical control. It is in the context of her narrative interviews with the recently bereaved that the notions of a good and a bad death emerge spontaneously as natural categories of thought. Given the conversational context of their emergence they are probably more accurately described as social, rather than as collective, repre-sentations. Their appearance, however, is constrained by the topic and the narrative nature of the conversation – the sequence of events culminating with their husband's funeral. In terms of the representa-tions involved the social is nested within the collective. The talk relates to the ritual, at least in part.

A corpus of talk about death and dying

The study is comparable to other recent innovative developments in the field of social psychology, like Billig's study *Talking of the Royal Family* (Billig 1992) and, more generally, the analysis of discourse. In Billig's study ordinary families in Middle England talked about an extraordinary family – the Monarchy. There was a pleasing harmony, here, between the locus (the family) and the focus (Royalty) of dis-cussion. The data that emerged were comparable to the data we obtain when using the focus group as our principal method of research. This is highly appropriate in relation to a theory like the theory of social representations since social representations form and are transformed in the course of conversations. In discourse analysis the relation between the discourse and the reality to which it refers is often quite tenuous, especially in cases where the theorist concerned rejects the idea that there is a reality which is distinct from the discourse about it. In Bradbury's study the discourse about death can be interpreted in terms of her observations concerning the work of the deathwork professionals. Her corpus of data concerns a corpse. This is why Chapter 5 (about the body) is central to the whole study. The trouble with Harry (Hitchcock's *The Trouble with Harry*, made in 1955) was that he was a corpse. The same is true of the central character in Karel Capek's novel *Meteor*.

That the corpse, in reality, was the central character in the drama emerged only at a late stage in the writing up of the original field-work. The two sets of data were analysed quite separately i.e. the participant observational studies of the deathwork professionals and the interviews with the sample of widows who had recently been bereaved. In regard to the arrangement of the funeral, if the funeral director was the provider of a service who was his/her client? Was it the widow? Or was it the corpse? The funeral director was clearly the Master of Ceremonies – and the study was a study of ceremonies and ritual – precisely because he had control of the corpse. Yet the study also included a discourse about the corpse – the discourse of the widows. It is this integration of two distinct sets of data which make Chapter 5 – about the body – pivotal to the whole study.

Professor Robert M. Farr
Department of Social Psychology
London School of Economics and Political Sciences

References

Billig, M. (1992) *Talking of the Royal Family*, London: Routledge.

Bloch, M. and Parry, J. (1982) *Death and the Regeneration of Life*, Cambridge: Cambridge University Press.

Culture and Psychology (1998) 4 (3), 275–429. Special Issue: One Hundred Years of Collective and Social Representatives. See especially the papers by Moscovici and Markova (pp. 371–410); Moscovici (pp. 411–428) and Farr (pp. 275–296).

Durkheim, E. (1898) 'Représentations individuelles et représentations collectives', *Revue de Metaphysique et de Morale* 6: 273–302.

Farr, R.M. (1978) 'On the social significance of artifacts in experimenting', *British Journal of Social and Clinical Psychology* 17: 299–306.

Glaser, B. and Strauss, A. (1965) *Awareness of Dying*, Chicago: Aldine.

Glaser, B. and Strauss, A. (1968) *A Time for Dying*, Chicago: Aldine.

Goffman, E. (1961) *Asylums: Essays on the Situation of Mental Patients and Other Inmates*, Harmondsworth: Penguin Books.

Jodelet, D. (1991) *Madness and Social Representations*, Brighton: Harvester Wheatsheaf.

Murchison, C.A. (ed.) (1935) *Handbook of Social Psychology*, Worcester, MA: Clark University Press.

Preface

Standing alone in a viewing chapel in a London funeral parlour almost a decade ago I was struck by the impossibility of coming to terms with the fact that one day I too would be lying in a spot-lit niche like the one before me. How could I become an inert object, not experiencing the scene, not there to tell the story? I have been studying death ever since. To be honest I cannot say that my efforts to come to terms with this aspect of life have been totally successful. Our mortality is a troubling matter. Yet my interest in the topic of death has been life enhancing. During my research I have had the privilege to come into contact with a great variety of people: the hassled casualty doctor; the underpaid intensive care nurse; the charming funeral director; the under-rated embalmer; the bereaved wife. They all agreed to share their knowledge with me about this natural part of our lives.

The data presented in the pages that follow were collected as part of a PhD thesis. In 1990 I went 'into the field' in London with the aim of presenting a social psychological study of death. Since I wrote the thesis my perspective on this data has changed somewhat. Since my first days in the library as a postgraduate, death has become a fashionable topic of research. Interdisciplinary conferences, new journals and a barrage of death-related books have made the old death-discoveries seem like old hat. It has not been the academic environment alone that has caused me to write the book afresh. The experiences of marriage, parenting, bereavement and psychoanalysis have changed me and have had an impact on the way in which I have interpreted and presented my findings.

Finally, I want to acknowledge that there is no such thing as academic distance when we come to study death. This was forcibly brought home to me recently while calmly reading a colleague's manuscript. In one passage I came across a husband's moving account of his wife's death in which he describes the appearance of her dead face; the woman, Ruth Picardie, was an old and dear university friend. The shock was such that I found myself gasping for breath. Suddenly the false veil of academic objectivity was torn away and I came face to face with all the pain and confusion that can be aroused by this most challenging of subjects.

Mary Bradbury
April 1999

Acknowledgements

A few months after the loss of their life's partner, twelve women volunteered to take part in a study about the experience of losing a husband and organizing his funeral. Their insights on the business of disposing of our beloved dead grace the pages that follow. I shall never forget the generosity of these women. I also want to thank the funeral director and the bereavement support group, Cruse, who helped to put me in contact with them. There were others who were involved in this study, who for obvious reasons I cannot name. I am grateful to those professionals who agreed to be interviewed and observed going about the daily business of their 'deathwork'. At times they were understandably nervous about how they would be portrayed – I appreciated their frankness.

The photographer Peter Rauter supplied the wonderful photographs that illustrate this book. Taking the photographs with Peter and his assistant Paul Blackshaw was an experience. I do not think I am going to forget in a hurry our day spent shooting in an embalming room. I wish to thank Jeremy West, of West and Coe, for throwing open his parlour doors to the cameras. Thanks also to Ian Hussein and Lynn Heath from the City of London Cemetery and Crematorium. T. Cribbs and Sons deserve a thank you for letting me photograph their wonderful horse-drawn hearse.

There is a thriving interdisciplinary academic community that has been brought together by a common interest in thanatology. I have been involved in conferences, books, journals, seminars and countless informal conversations with a group of anthropologists, historians, psychologists and sociologists who have all shared a passion for understanding aspects of our mortality. With pleasure I acknowledge the intellectual debt I owe to David Clark, David Field, Jenny Hockey, Glennys Howarth, Ralph Houbrooke, Peter Jupp, Jeanne Katz, Lindsey Prior, Ruth Richardson, Neil Small and Tony Walter. I would also like to thank Ken Elliot and Philip Gore for their valuable professional advice.

My supervisors played a central role in the development of the theory and methodology of the thesis that forms the backbone of this book. I always remember with a smile Bram Oppenheim's unflagging enthusiasm for his 'death supervisions' with me. Many of the ideas in this book originally came from him. After Bram's retirement, Robert Farr took over, providing much inspiration and support. Robert introduced me to Serge Moscovici and the theory of social representations. I want to thank him for all of his help. I am delighted and touched that he has written the foreword. My friend Vanessa Cragnow, the departmental secretary, deserves a big thank you for her endless support and hope.

I have noticed that people always thank their editor for being patient. Now I know why. The release of this particular book faced two hefty delays called baby Joe and baby Ellie and I was particularly thankful that I had such an understanding person in Heather Gibson. Thanks also to Fiona Bailey for being such a calm and helpful senior editorial assistant once the book got on its way.

Thanks go to Robert Farr, Katy Gardner, Esther Selsdon and my parents, Isobel and Robert Bradbury, for their helpful comments about the manuscript. Hélène Joffe deserves credit for helping me with the title. In fact there would be no manuscript to read or titles to construct if it had not been for the kindness of Rebecca Mascarenhas who, prior to my getting ESRC funding, supported me in the first year of my PhD.

The writing of a book inevitably draws in the family. Joe still looks suspicious when I go near my iMac. In addition to shouldering a heavy load of childcare my husband, Mark Swartzentruber, put many, many hours of work into the production of this book. Finally, I have chosen to dedicate this book to my dear parents because I wanted to thank them for bringing me up to think I could do anything, even study death.

God forbid that we get something wrong. It is just mortifying.

(Funeral Director)

Introduction

An analysis of contemporary deathways

The last decade of the twentieth century has witnessed a quiet revolution in our relationship with mortality. We are currently experiencing dramatic changes in demographic patterns as people live longer and take more time to die. Death hidden and denied has become death discussed and analysed and this book is part of that 'chatter'. With the close of the modern era the privatization and sequestration of death that had become the mantra of social scientists has slowly been eroded by a new openness. In many ways I was lucky to witness this moment of social change and the research that forms the basis for this book represents a snapshot of this extraordinary period. At times I came across deathways that were typical of those descriptions of death and dying made nearly thirty years earlier by sociologists such as Glaser and Strauss where people's experience of dying and of being bereaved were dominated by the medical model and expressed a deep unease with our mortality. In contrast, there were occasions in which I found myself surprised by lay social innovators who tackled death head on, negotiated with medical practitioners, rejected conventional funerals and generally seemed to be inordinately interested in the business of death, dying and bereavement.

I spent many months observing, participating and interviewing people involved in the care of the dying and the disposal of the dead. I also interviewed women who had lost their husband some months previously. My anthropological training had led me to expect that I would not find anything that remotely approached a proper mortuary ritual in contemporary London. If anything, my tentative research hypotheses were drawn up to describe a greedy industry, empty rituals, hollow customs and pathologically grieving customers. Fortunately, the qualitative nature of the study allowed me to be surprised. I stumbled on vibrant social customs and vivid accounts of ritual participation: a shrine, complete with an old answerphone tape which contained the dear deceased's voice; letters of condolence that flooded the doormat of a bereaved person; an exotic personal rite in which the ashes were distributed according to the strict pre-death instructions of the deceased; weekly trips to adorn a carefully chosen and lovingly maintained memorial. In the depth of a metropolitan city I came across rites of passage in which the participants underwent transformations. I found survivors who believed in an afterlife which was peopled with ancestors, ghosts and even 'cells of the dead' which, apparently, circle in the ether.

An essential component of this ritual process is the discourse that surrounds death. In this book, I explore the ways in which we talk about death in terms of it being a good or bad, natural or unnatural event. Using the social psychological theory of social representations, I identified three existing representations of the 'good death'. These representations work as powerful social norms, presenting the survivors with 'acceptable' ways of talking about death. Deaths were explained as being good because they were 'spiritual', because they conformed to an idealized vision of a medically controlled event or, conversely, because they were seen to be rejecting what is increasingly viewed as an over-interventionist approach to dying. An analysis of these representations demonstrates that they do not offer us the opportunity of obtaining 'good death recipes' in which we merely have to add the right mix of ingredients in order to get the desired result. Indeed, I found myself being presented with an ever-changing kaleidoscope of descriptions of death in which all three representations of death were layered on top of one another.

The apparently arbitrary character of the split between good and bad or natural and unnatural does not imply that they do not have an important role to play, however. Our talk about death has a very real impact on how we die, what we do with our dead and how we experience our bereavements. As a social psychologist I was particularly interested to explore the interactions between rituals, customs and representations – that strange and shadowy world in which a representation of, say, the good medical death becomes anchored and objectified in an embalmer's efforts to make a corpse look as if it is asleep.

My research revealed how theories generated in the academic community filter down to the lay population. I found that 'scientific' knowledge can become distorted in the process of dissemination by the mass media. My respondents were quick to inform me about their knowledge of the stage–phase models of grieving. But these lay models seemed to be mutant beasts. People talked to me of the necessity of working through every stage in sequence, they pondered on their apparent failure to 'get out of the anger stage' and shared their fears that their grief would turn 'unhealthy'. Their unique experiences of loss were being conventualized by social representations of healthy grief.

There are eight chapters in this book. The first two deal with the theory and methodology used in a social psychological study of death. In addition to a brief introduction to the theory of social representations, the opening chapter attempts to contextualize current representations of death by providing a social historical overview of the British funeral. The chapter that follows outlines the methods used in the data-collection process. Inspired by classic volumes such as *When Prophecy Fails* (Festinger *et al.* 1956) I have given a thorough ethnographic account of my days in the field and the business of analysing the data.

Disposing of a body in contemporary Western society is extraordinarily complicated and in Chapters 3 and 4 I give a description of what we currently do with our dead. The death system is loosely separated into four domains through which the survivors and the deceased pass as they progress along the route towards memorialization. The medical and bureaucratic aspects of death are described in the first of these twin chapters. This is a time in which the survivors find themselves making visits to hospitals, patients' affairs rooms and register offices; they are interviewed, they pick up forms and they answer questions. The next chapter turns to the commercial and ritual face of contemporary death. Now it is the turn of the funeral director, the clergyman or woman and the wonderfully named 'memorial counsellor' to take control of the grieving 'client'. It is in this domain that many people find themselves unexpectedly making purchases; to their mild surprise they have become consumers.

In Chapter 5 I re-examine the death system through anthropological glasses, exploring the body's role in structuring our ritual responses to death. Indeed, the repeated re-presentation of the pseudo-medically manipulated corpse is a striking characteristic of contemporary Western mortuary rites. Reinterpreting this death process, I argue that many of the activities that appear to be rational, such as embalming, also have an expressive role. Much is being said about life, death and society itself when we pump pink formaldehyde into a corpse's arteries, sew its mouth shut and file its nails.

The next two chapters focus on ways in which we represent death and loss. Drawing on social historical and anthropological theories of the good death and applying them to my own data, Chapter 6 describes social representations of the good natural, medical or sacred death. I explore the ways in which we anchor the unfamiliar and unknown in the familiar and hackneyed phrase 'it was a good death'. The chapter closes with a discussion of the ways in which the cancer death appears to provide us with 'good death ingredients' and how this 'ideal' may fail to be realized. Chapter 7 starts with a critique of conventional models of grief as a disease. I draw attention to the dichotomization of loss into healthy and unhealthy reactions and discuss the parallels that this opposition into desirable and undesirable outcomes has with the process of labelling a death as either good or bad. I also argue that the de-socialized model of grief as a solely individual phenomenon fails to take into account the social nature of mind. I suggest that by using Mead we can gain a better understanding of cross-cultural and historical differences in the nature of grief. This socialized conception of loss also helps us to understand the almost universal practice of memorialization in which the survivors conduct postmortem relationships with the dead.

The book closes with a chapter in which I present the merits of adopting a social psychological perspective on death. Making use of Mead and Moscovici I call for a focus on culture in which language, custom, ritual, science and the media are interwoven to produce a rite of passage that is both different and the same as those death practices of other cultures, past and present.

1 The study of death

A social psychological approach

Death in a city

Driving though London recently on a busy working day I came across a funeral cortège sedately making its way to the local crematorium: shiny black hearse, flowers, bearers and the coffin. Bunched up behind the limousines was a long trail of London traffic which had been forced to adopt this morbid pace. No one overtook the cortège, although there were plenty of opportunities to do so. It is often said that death is hidden in contemporary society, but I am not so sure. As I trundled along behind the mourners I saw a funeral parlour I had failed to notice before and a signpost to the crematorium. If we look, we can see that the business of disposing of the dead is part of the urban landscape. My slow drive behind a funeral made me aware of this other world, unnoticed in the business of day-to-day life.

Any culture is faced with certain physical, metaphysical and social challenges when someone dies. In this book I look at the British response to death in an urban environment at the beginning of the 1990s. I chose to go into the field and spent months observing, participating and interviewing. Our death practices take place in a variety of sites: hospital, hospice, home, funeral parlour, crematorium and cemetery. I moved from site to site, following the corpse's progress along our relatively lengthy death routes. On the basis of this qualitative study I have found myself emphasizing both continuity and change. Within the same funeral we can find a heady mix of horse-drawn hearses and marble memorial stones, alongside the playing of an Elvis song in a committal service.

The study of death can be approached in many ways. We can describe the process of dying, reveal the inequalities in demographic patterns of mortality, discuss the ethical debates raging around the point of death, attempt to describe the feelings of the bereaved, examine the institutions that deal with the dying and the dead or analyse mortuary rituals. In the past these topics have been divided into separate and discrete chunks. For example, broadly speaking, the study of rituals has become the domain of social anthropologists; the study of grief, the property of psychologists. However, it is rarely possible or desirable to explore an aspect of death in isolation. If we are describing a death ritual we should also discuss the sentiments of the participants. The traditional boundaries that meant, for example, that sociologists wandered around hospitals and hospices observing the day-to-day work that went on while psychiatrists and psychologists interviewed grieving widows, are beginning to collapse. Many studies are breaking new ground. For example, Attig (1996), a philosopher, and Davies (1997), a theologian, both offer refreshing perspectives on the subject of grief and mourning.

Remaining within a sociological tradition of social psychology I make use of Moscovici's (1984a) theory of social representations and draw extensively on the work that came out of the 'Chicago School' (Mead 1934; Goffman 1959). This has certain repercussions. Adopting an essentially social view of mind and personhood I am turning my back on individual models of grief and mourning. I want to bring into focus the construction of representations of death and loss through social interaction. In order to understand this process I am going to stray into the fields of social anthropology and sociology.

When we come to explore broad topics such as health, illness or death, this inclusive stance is necessary. Certainly, Radley (1994), one of the rare social psychologists who embraces a qualitative approach, found this to be the case in his analysis of health and illness; in this instance, he reviews medical sociology, health psychology and medical anthropology. As Radley notes 'when we try to make sense of illness we find that we are, often unintentionally, also making sense of life, and perhaps ourselves as well' (1994: preface).

I was interested in studying death practices in a contemporary urban setting. I wanted to look at what people do and what people feel. As a consequence, I found myself facing the challenge of integrating the overlapping areas of grief, mourning, mortuary rituals, the institutions that deal with death and the industry that makes its profits from the dead. At first I felt in a privileged position as a social psychologist. The very name of my discipline holds the hope for a successful fusion of mind and culture. Although social psychology would appear to be ideally suited to the task of marrying public action with private emotion, when I came to review the social psychological literature on death and dying I was to be disappointed. Social psychology has been surprisingly quiet on the subject of death. Some explanation for this can be found in the discipline's history, which is briefly described at the end of this chapter.

Social history

Social representations theory has an appreciation not only of culture but also of history. To unravel our current representations of death expressed in language, cultural artefacts and behaviour it is crucial to place them in a historical context. Trying to arrive at an understanding of contemporary representations of death and loss without an appreciation of their underlying history which lies behind would be as pointless as undertaking psychoanalysis without talking about our past.

Dying and bereavement are difficult things to contemplate and it comes as no surprise that it is slightly easier when we create a sense of distance. Death in other eras and cultures can be interesting rather than threatening. Elias warns the unwary against looking 'mistrustfully at the bad present in the name of a better past' (1985: 12). In similar vein, Hockey (1996) looks at the ways in which the death rituals of our past and those of non-industrial cultures have been interpreted by social scientists interested in grief work. In our current therapy-orientated culture the multifunctional nature of participation in ritual is often denied in favour of a model in which ritual acts are seen only as a conduit for the expression of emotions. However, in reality, mortuary rituals are often more caught up in the expression of wealth and the distribution of power. Drawing on the dichotomy between 'nature' and 'science' Hockey argues that there has been an assumption expressed in both ethnographic accounts and the bereavement literature that pre-industrial community-based deathways are in some way superior to those of our modern-day rational practices. As she points out, there is no evidence to support the thesis that traditional death practices were in any way 'better', or more therapeutic, for the participants, giving them unique access to healthy, natural responses to death. In the account of pre-industrial Britain that follows it is valuable to keep Elias's and Hockey's points in mind.

In the last 200 years the processes of dying and disposal have undergone a transformation. The use of professionals to prepare the corpse and the practice of cremation are both examples of relatively recent innovations. Houlbrooke (1989) identifies the Victorian era in Great Britain as the time when social practices and attitudes changed most dramatically. He attempts to outline some of the social changes

in the years before that contributed to this and identifies the following: the reformation, the rise of the natural sciences, the secular
climate of opinion and the increasing influence of the medical profession. Other authors have argued that changing attitudes towards
death can be explained by the rise of individualism in the Western
world (Ariès 1974, 1983; Gittings 1984). Houlbrooke (1989)
questions the utility of citing such a global cause because, in practice,
it is difficult to identify the impact of 'individualism' let alone define it.

In the early nineteenth century British 'funerals' were composite
rituals which took place over several days and the locus of control lay
with the community (Richardson 1989). People usually died at home
in the company of family members, although as Elias (1985) is quick
to point out, we should be wary of idealizing such deaths for the social
nature of these events may have had very little to do with the
acceptance of death or, for that matter, close family ties. In conditions
of overcrowding it may have been rather difficult to find a room in
which one could die on one's own.

> Everyone is familiar with pictures from earlier periods, showing
> how whole families – women, men and children – gather around
> the bed of a dying matri- or patriarch. That may be a romantic
> idealisation. Families in that situation may often have been scorn-
> ful, brutal and cold. Rich people perhaps did not always die
> quickly enough for their heirs. Poor people may have lain in their
> filth and starved.
>
> (Elias 1985: 75)

After a death, female family members would prepare the corpse,
helped by the neighbourhood layers-out, women who informally
helped in the tasks of both birth and death. Adams (1993) provides
a fascinating account of female community layers-out in the working-
class area of Coventry in the interwar years and notes that care of the
dead was not organized in terms of kinship or male work, but was
characterized 'by the pattern of informal care organised by the women
in response to their shared experience of economic insecurity and
poverty, the absence of public welfare and the imperative to maintain
self respect' (1993: 149). These women were often paid in kind for
their work. The layer-out possessed skills and exercised her arts in a
flexible and varied way. She adapted to circumstances and played
things by ear, sensitive to the needs of the bereaved-to-be or bereaved
family. This behaviour stands in contrast to the routinized and planned
procedures that are characteristic of more modern institutions. These

'tidy' ladies made every effort to make the body presentable for family and friends. They washed the body and plugged orifices. The legs were straightened, arms folded across the chest or stomach and the eyes and mouth closed. The corpse's hair was brushed and combed. It would often receive a manicure or a shave. The body would then be dressed in a white shroud and, possibly, wrapped up in a 'winding sheet' that left the face exposed until the point of burial (Richardson 1988: 17). Adams (1993), calling attention to the old tradition of tightly wrapping both new-borns and corpses, notes the close similarities between the ways of treating those entering and those exiting our society.

Close relatives would observe the tradition of 'watching the dead' until the day of burial, which was often preceded by a rather festive and noisy wake (Richardson 1988: 22). Meanwhile grieving friends and relatives would visit and view the body over the next day or so to pay their last respects. During this time the layer-out would continue to be active in helping the family, making cakes and sandwiches and even lending crockery (Adams 1993). If the family could afford it, a local carpenter would make a coffin. Alternatively the body would be simply buried in its winding sheet (Richardson 1988: 20). Providing there were no reasons, such as suicide, to preclude burial in conse-crated ground the deceased would be carried to the graveyard for burial, followed by the mourners.

The very wealthy and the very poor, however, could expect quite different funerals. Those who died in poverty had their body uncer-emoniously dumped in a communal grave pit on the edge of the graveyard. In contrast, aristocratic families often spent vast quantities of money on heraldic funerals. These were elaborate, meticulously organized and fantastically expensive affairs.

Aspirations of conspicuous consumption notwithstanding, these mortuary rituals served the serious business of marking the passage from the world of the living to the world of the dead. Almost every aspect of these early funerals was imbued with some kind of sacred, spiritual or, at the very least, superstitious symbolic meaning. For example, Richardson (1988: 26) notes how rumbustious wakes were believed to ward off evil spirits. In similar vein it was believed that opening windows or doors allowed the soul to escape. Clocks were stopped, mirrors were turned against the wall and fires were extin-guished. These customs were full of symbolic meaning in the hour of death (Richardson 1988: 27). Funerals were multifunctional. Not only did the various customary and ritual observances help to allay fears of being haunted by homeless and malicious spirits, but they also facilitated the redistribution of goods, roles and statuses among the surviving community. Most importantly, these funerals expressed the community's belief that death leads to regeneration and rebirth.

Death and medical science

Benoliel and Degner (1995) note that before the establishment of modern medicine, patterns of living and of dying were quite different. Life was less predictable. Infant mortality was high and women often died in childbirth. The causes of most deaths then, such as influenza, pneumonia and tuberculosis, are now relatively easy to contain and treat (for a fuller discussion, see Stillion 1995). Even if a person was suffering from cancer it would often be an attack of pneumonia that would kill them.

As the science of medicine became established the promise of increased longevity or, at the very least, of reduced pain made the presence of a doctor at the point of death more common. The administration of opiates meant that it was possible to die in a relatively pain-free state. So, providing the patients could afford the doctor and the drugs, they could aspire to die as if in sleep. Porter (1989), in his analysis of the role of the doctor in the nineteenth century, suggests that, rather than viewing disease and death as acts of God, doctors came to see disease as a natural cause of death. It therefore became acceptable for them to 'manage' the death bed. Dying in a drug-induced unconscious state was seen as an ideal. This stands in contrast to the image of the good death of earlier centuries in which the dying remained conscious and interactive to the end (Beier 1989). For the burgeoning middle classes with money to spend, dying, traditionally a sacred moment, was becoming a secular activity that was dominated by a new class of professionals. Priests, who used to play a central role in the drama of dying, were being usurped by the doctor. The doctor became the person 'to step in between the individual and their death' (Hockey 1990: 71).

The influence of the medical sciences on our death rites did not stop at the moment of death. This new science needed bodies for research purposes. In a wonderful study, Richardson (1988) has traced the impact of the anatomists on both our mortuary rituals and our representations of death. Although mortality rates were high in the eighteenth and nineteenth centuries, bodies for dissection were in short supply. Dissection was viewed with great distrust as people grappled with the theological complexities of the link between the state of the body and the state of the soul. As Richardson notes (1988: 32), dissection was viewed as a form of punishment, 'a fate worse than death'. Only those who had died the most shameful of deaths were suitable candidates for dissection. Many bodies came from the hangman's noose.

It did not take long for the criminal classes to realize that a good income could be obtained through the unpleasant task of exhuming the newly and not-so-newly dead. Richardson notes that while the penalties for grave-robbing were relatively lenient, for the times, this was still a dangerous occupation; one would not want to be found by an angry mob. Generally the resurrectionists favoured robbing paupers' graves: large pits into which many bodies were piled (Richardson 1988: 60).

During the last decades of the eighteenth century fresh or anatomically unusual corpses could command handsome prices (Richardson 1988: 58). Monetary value was thus attached to the body for the first time (Richardson 1988: 52).

> Corpses were bought and sold, they were touted, priced, haggled over, negotiated for, discussed in terms of supply and demand, delivered, imported, exported, transported. Human bodies were compressed into boxes, packed in sawdust, packed in hay, trussed up in sacks, roped up like hams, sewn in canvas, packed in cases, casks, barrels, crates and hampers; salted, pickled or injected with preservative. They were carried in carts and waggons, in barrows and steam-boats; manhandled, damaged in transit, and hidden under loads of vegetables. They were stored in cellars and on quays. Human bodies were dismembered and sold in pieces, or measured and sold by the inch.
>
> (Richardson 1988: 72)

Body-snatching caught the popular imagination and rich and poor alike lived in great fear of a surgeon's illegal post-mortem. The nation appeared to exist in a state of near hysteria regarding this emotive topic. Death practices underwent subtle alterations in response to this perceived threat. An iron coffin was patented which, it was claimed, could not be opened by body-snatchers; others chose thick wood coffins; straw and sticks were added to soil in order to clog the grave-digger's spade; bodies were buried deep; tombstone and vault design was defensive as well as decorative; grave sites were guarded at night by watchmen (Richardson 1988).

In 1828 the protest against body-snatching and the practices of the anatomists reached new heights when it was discovered that two individuals from Edinburgh called Burke and Hare had been murdering poor and vulnerable citizens to supply the local medical school. Although such an event had been predicted for some time, there was a national outcry (Richardson 1988: 133). In response to public demand the government had already been working on a select committee report on anatomy. This insensitive report suggested that the bodies of those who died in poverty, in workhouses, could be dissected. Richardson notes that, given the general population's highly negative view of dissection, the government was, in effect, penalizing the poor. In response to the threat of such a terrifying end, the working classes set up burial societies in which members contributed money for their future funerals (Richardson 1988: 277). Richardson suggests that the working-class's emphasis on saving money for 'a proper funeral' dates back to these times. As a public relations exercise, it would appear that both the anatomy schools and the government were guilty of appalling misjudgement. Implementing the Anatomy Act of 1832 was fraught with administrative and bureaucratic hurdles. It never helped to alleviate the constant shortage of corpses for dissection. Nevertheless, as people began to enjoy the benefits of medicine, dissection did gradually gain acceptance in the general population. Nowadays, the supply is met through personal bequests by members of the public (see Richardson 1995).

A fledgling industry

In an increasingly secular, rationalist and scientific climate of thought, many beliefs that had been accepted for centuries were open to scrutiny. During the Victorian era a new urban middle class became a force in English society. These educated and articulate people were faced with many innovations in thought and practice. It is no surprise, therefore, that in this environment there were so many radical transformations in British deathways.

The aspiring middle class was keen to emulate the upper class. They appropriated the black ribbons and feathers and the yards of crêpe and silk, the use of which dated back to the ancient heraldic rites. A whole industry was founded on this fashion for mourning. Funerals provided a perfect, if rather late, opportunity to display one's spending power.

> Manifest in the increasingly commercialised trappings of death, the funeral came to be the rite of passage *par excellence* by which to assert financial and social position – a secular last judgement which had as its goal the exhibition of worldly respectability.
>
> (Richardson 1988: 272)

Highly restrictive female mourning practices developed during this time. If a family member died, the close female relatives were expected to remain in deep mourning for many months. Incapacitating family members for the purposes of mourning was yet another way of expressing one's wealth; the family demonstrated that it could afford the luxury of non-productive persons. Thus, during the Victorian era, women's traditionally active roles at the death bed were replaced by more passive roles.

While the body had always been a powerful symbolic object – alive or dead – in Victorian England it began to assume an untouchable quality. Many families discarded the old female role of laying out their dead. With the combination of class consciousness, which made it undesirable to fraternize with common 'deathwives' and an increasing squeamishness towards the body, it comes as no surprise that well-to-do people felt it more seemly to leave the intimate tasks involved in laying-out to male professionals (Morely 1971). In working-class areas the move away from informal patterns of care in which specific members of the community could be approached to help with the laying-out of the dead took longer to disintegrate (Adams 1993). At the moment of birth a similar revolution in roles was taking place. The Midwives Act of 1902 in which local authorities found themselves accountable for all practising midwives in their areas had the rapid effect of pushing out of practice any women who had not undertaken formal training. Meanwhile, in the more prosperous circles it became fashionable to dispense with the traditional female midwife in favour of a male *coucheur*.

This professionalization of death was to have profound repercussions on our experience of bereavement. In these shifts we can see how death was removed from the domain of the family. Increasingly women were being excluded from the social organization of death. The use of male professionals did not stop with the laying-out of the dead; contemporary funerals of the time became so complicated that it soon became necessary to hand over the organization of the funeral to the newly empowered undertakers. In an analysis of the development of funeral firms in East Kent, Gore (1992) notes how carpenters found themselves adopting this specialist role by public demand. The new undertakers could charge a great deal for their services. Although many people would have felt some relief in being able to hand the business of disposing of the dead to another person, Richardson believes that the use of such professionals represented an 'invasion of commerce into the rite of passage' (Richardson 1988: 4). Gradually, with the introduction of medical, bureaucratic and commercial concerns, the space between death and burial expanded.

A crisis in the disposal of the dead

In Britain's cities, conditions for the working classes were unsanitary and cramped. The mortality rate was high and it was not long before urban graveyards also began to be overcrowded. There were fears for public health. In the 1830s the Chadwick report on the state of London's churchyards exposed a terrible state of affairs. Porter (1994) quotes Chadwick 'on spaces of ground that do not exceed 203 acres, closely surrounded by the abodes of the living, 20,000 adults and nearly 30,000 youths and children are every year imperfectly interred'. The whole burial ground in Russell Court was raised several feet by burials and was, according to Chadwick, a 'mass of corruption' (Porter 1994: 273). Matters took a turn for the worse when the cholera outbreak of 1831 claimed many thousands of lives. By the autumn of that year alone 5000 people had already died (Porter 1994).

In cities such as London, the combination of a fear of body-snatching (always more common in graveyards close to Anatomy Schools (Richardson 1988)) and the unsavoury state of most churchyards made it desirable to bury one's dead elsewhere. For those that could afford it, rural burial seemed an attractive option. In response to this demand certain entrepreneurs opened joint-stock cemeteries on the outskirts of the major cities. A good example of one of these once-rural cemeteries is Highgate Cemetery in North London, opened in 1839. Burial in such cemeteries was expensive. In an atmosphere of social one-up-manship and freedom from the constraints of the church, secular themes for monuments began to dominate. In many London cemeteries we see nubile nymphs, weeping women and Egyptian and Grecian tombs. For those who could not afford such extravagances the problems of post-mortem urban overcrowding continued to be pressing and worrisome. In 1850 and 1852 the Burial Acts passed responsibility for finding land for burial from the religious authorities to local authorities.

There were alternatives to burial. In the 1870s Sir Henry Thompson advocated cremation of the dead as a modern, scientific, hygienic and space-saving option. As Leaney has noted (1989) much of the rhetoric employed by the cremationists emphasized a feeling of revulsion towards the decaying corpse and the barbarism in letting it decay in the soil compared with the quick return to nature provided by cremation. The cremationist movement was formed in 1874 with

Sir Henry as its president. There was a great deal of discussion in the press and resistance was widespread. Some objections were based on common sense. For example, people argued that evidence of possible foul play would be destroyed in the cremators; this led to changes in medical certification that have continued to this day. Most concern, however, seems to have been focused on a debate about the resurrection of the body. Although the immortal soul should, in theory, not be affected by the mode of disposal, age-old anxieties about resurrection were still prevalent.

In 1884 the cremation of the dead was legally recognized. Various designs of cremators were discussed. In 1885 the first crematorium was opened in Woking, Surrey; three bodies were cremated that year (Davies 1997). The first local-authority-owned crematorium was opened eight years later. Ancient religious trappings, traditionally part of the burial rite, were deliberately incorporated in this innovative custom. Committal rooms were designed to look like churches, and early cremators were placed underground, so that the coffin could sink from the public space to the lower level. These efforts of ritual engineering were not always wholly successful and may help to explain why, a century later, the cremation ceremony can still at times feel contrived.

Cremation was not popular at first. Indeed, representations of death and loss had to undergo quite dramatic transformations in order to encompass this alien and strange form of disposal. The impetus for such changes was provided by the two World Wars. Cannadine (1981) provides a fascinating exploration of changes in representations of death resulting from the First World War. Referring to the period immediately after the First World War he notes:

> Death had become so ubiquitous and tragic, and grief so widespread and overwhelming, that even those remaining Victorian rituals – probably never effective even in the mid-nineteenth century – were now recognised as being inadequate, superfluous and irrelevant.
>
> (Cannadine 1981: 218)

So although the dead were still being buried, one could detect changes in death rites resulting from the two world wars. In the context of the slaughter of the First World War, the idea of staging showy, expensive funerals or of displaying hysterical and unrelenting grief seemed inappropriate. In the Second World War the social pressure to display a stoic reaction on losing close friends and family was consolidated.

Showing a 'brave face' and keeping 'a stiff upper lip' were positively sanctioned actions and mourners were congratulated on their fortitude. The stage was set for the 'death denying' culture of the 1950s and 1960s. The cremation ceremony – secular, quick and hidden out of sight – peculiarly suited this modern environment of thought and behaviour.

In 1939, fewer than 4 per cent of funerals were cremations. By 1944, the rate had crept up to 7 per cent (Jupp 1993). By the early 1950s local authorities were finding that the burial of the dead was an expensive undertaking, as early cemeteries began to fill and new land had to be found. Keen to develop and encourage a less expensive option, many local authorities built crematoria and kept the fees low. This appears to have been a successful strategy. By the 1960s half the population chose to cremate their dead. The figure currently stands at about 70 per cent.

Davies (1997) suggests that cremation's current popularity can partly be explained by its non-denominational character. Most memorial chapels in crematoria will remove or reinstate religious symbols as requested. The profits from cremation go to a neutral body, too, as most crematoria are owned by local authorities. Williams (1990) has also noted that cremation also fits in nicely with the atheist belief in the finality of death.

Another innovation was the practice of embalming which first found its way to British shores from the United States at the turn of the century. Embalming was slow to catch on and, until recently, British embalming practices were somewhat crude in comparison to the skills and effort put into the presentation of the dead in the United States. Embalming the dead in Britain became more desirable as the waiting period between cremation or burial and death increased to seven days or more under the pressures of numbers and as a result of increasingly complicated bureaucracy. In the winter months cemeteries and crematoria are overbooked and relatives may have to wait two weeks for the committal service. Another reason why undertakers have been keen to get the British public to embalm their dead was that it represented yet another specialized, 'professional', skill. This was something they could do for the body while they looked after it. It also justified an increase in the fee.

It is clear that British mortuary rites have undergone many changes in the last couple of centuries. Medical science occupies the centre stage in both the process of dying and the processing of the dead. In an increasingly secular society, less importance is placed on the fate of the soul. The clergy are being slowly shunted out of British death rites.

Meanwhile, the new professional class of funeral directors, as they have come to be called, have made themselves indispensable as the women who knew how to lay-out the dead have died themselves. This domestic skill is now almost completely lost. Finally, changes in the ways that we dispose of our dead have meant that we have had to assimilate embalming and cremation. Current representations of death are grounded in this social history.

I now wish to lay the theoretical foundations for the data presented in the subsequent chapters. In the remaining part of this chapter I will introduce the theory of social representations. The theory of social representations represents something of a departure from mainstream social psychology and for this reason I think it is helpful to give some background to the context in which it developed. This can be achieved by looking at social psychology's brief lifespan and in the section that follows I will give an overview of the discipline's 50-year history.

Social representations theory: a social psychological approach

Wundt is largely remembered as the founder of the science of experimental psychology, but he also developed a *Völkerpsychologie* (1900–20), in which the objects of study were language, religion, customs, myth, magic and cognate phenomena (Farr 1983, 1996). So culture was part of psychology. Both Wundt's laboratory science and his *Völkerpsychologie* were 'imported' to North America, but, Farr argues, it was the former that dominated.

Making use of Marková's (1982) thesis concerning the social Hegelian and the non-social Cartesian paradigms in philosophy, Farr (1996) suggests that the 'virus of individualism' inherited from Cartesianism 'infected' psychology. The Cartesian inheritance in psychology is a mental, introspective philosophy of the self and a behavioural science of the other. When psychology rejected mentalism in favour of behaviourism it never freed itself of Cartesian dualism, but merely switched the focus of study from the self to the other. The same fate seems to have befallen social psychology, which has remained social in name only. Keen to align itself to the natural sciences, modern social psychology became a science of human behaviour. Foremost of the reductionists was F. H. Allport who, in 1924, with the publication of his volume *Social Psychology*, turned the discipline into a behavioural and experimental science. From there on the social was individualized. Allport believed that we can understand the collective in terms of the individual – society is simply made up of groups of individuals. Politics played a part in this too. During the cold war researchers were more likely to get funding for the behavioural sciences than for the social sciences as those who supplied the funding did not distinguish between the social sciences and socialism (Farr 1996).

There were pockets of resistance. The great work of Mead in Chicago is an example. Mead spent his life attempting to understand the balance between the individual's mind and the society in which they live. Drawing on Wundt's *Völkerspsychologie* (1900–20) and the work of Darwin, Mead 'interpolated self between mind and society' (Farr 1996: 54) and in the process he naturalized the mind.

> [Mead] demonstrated the dialectical nature of the relationship between the individual and society. Individualisation is the outcome of socialisation and not its antithesis. The self in humans needs to be understood both phylogenetically, in terms of the evolution of the species, and ontogenetically, in terms of the development of each individual member of the species.
>
> (Farr 1996: 54)

For Mead, mind was the product of language. 'Mind arises through communication by a conversation of gestures in a social process or context of experience – not communication through mind' (Mead 1934: 50). Therefore thinking is also a social activity, a kind of conversation held with oneself. As a pragmatist philosopher, Mead fought against dualisms, such as the split between self and other, that Descartes had introduced into philosophy. Marková (1987) notes how Mead showed that self emerges from social interaction. We become an object to ourselves simply by assuming the role of the other with regard to ourselves; thus, 'the nature of consciousness in humans is an awareness of self in relation to others. Consciousness is thus an inherently social process' (Farr 1996: 67).

Farr (1996) notes that Mead was repudiated by the positivists in psychology and his research findings were given little attention in the histories written about the discipline (Allport 1954) or in handbooks (Lindzey 1954; Lindzey and Aronson 1968, 1985). From this historical perspective we can begin to understand the reason why so little truly social research has been undertaken by social psychologists in the last few decades, particularly in North America. In the psychological traditions of social psychology the study of culture and of society has been unfashionable for years. Without an understanding of, and sympathy for, culture, the study of death remains one-dimensional.

The only option available is to research individual behavioural responses to death, i.e. to study the grief reaction.

The theory of social representations also belongs to the sociological tradition of social psychology. This relatively new theory, founded by Moscovici (1984a), hails from France. It provides us with the exciting opportunity of reintroducing culture to the discipline of psychology.

The theory of social representations

They do not represent simply 'opinions about', 'images of' or 'attitudes towards' but 'theories' or 'branches of knowledge' in their own right, for the discovery and organisation of reality . . . Systems of values, ideas and practices with a twofold function; first, to establish an order which will enable individuals to orientate themselves in their material and social world and to master it; secondly, to enable communication to take place among members of a community by providing them with a code for social exchange and a code for naming and classifying unambiguously the various aspects of their world and their individual and group history.

(Moscovici in foreword to Herzlich 1973: xiii)

Moscovici envisioned representations as social constructions that form an 'environment of thought'. This environment of thought shapes our perceptions and conceptions of an object. So what we perceive in the world is a socially constructed reality held within certain cultural and historical boundaries. Moscovici (1985) has always been loath to constrain these explanatory models of our world – these ways of seeing and thinking – through the use of operational definitions. However, the lack of clear definitions of 'social representations' has been criticized (Hewstone 1985; Potter and Litton 1985; Purkhardt 1991). This lack of definition has allowed a range of interpretations of the meaning of 'social' and 'representation'.

Certain problems have probably stemmed from the translation of the term from French to English. Drawing on Harré (1984) and Purkhardt (1993), I have taken the meaning of 'social' to mean the transmission and creation of representations and the social reality created by representations. Alternative definitions, such as the object being represented, the social milieu within which representations arise, or the shared character of representations, appear to underestimate the truly social meaning of this act of representing the world. Turning to 'representation' I agree with Harré (1984) who suggests that, rather than translating the French '*représentation*' to the English meaning of a likeness or copy, we should translate the word as 'version'.

> What goes on in people's minds when they are faced with life's great enigmas such as illness, our bodies, our origins, knowledge, death, etc.? How do systems of social representations, this imposing heritage that turns us into active participants in society even without our being aware of it, how do these systems come into being and then evolve? These are questions historians and anthropologists try to answer, and they are relevant even for us as social psychologists.
>
> (Moscovici 1984b: 941)

As Farr (1993) points out, the diffusion of social representations' theory into the English speaking world has, until recently, been slow. Fortunately, some fine empirical studies have made it across the channel, such as Herzlich's (1973) study of the social representations of health and illness among town and country folk, Chombart de Lauwe's (1984) study of the social representations of childhood and Jodelet's (1991) study of representations of mental illness. At last British studies are beginning to surface, too. Notable among these is Joffe's (1999) work with current social representations of risk, with reference to HIV.

Moscovici identified various 'functions' of representations: to construct our reality, facilitate communication and social interaction, demarcate and consolidate groups, aid the formation of social identity, serve in the process of socialization and, finally, make the unfamiliar familiar. Representations perform these functions by the process of anchoring, in which we use classification and naming to give a new object meaning, and objectification, in which we make the unfamiliar familiar by objectifying it (Purkhardt 1991).

Moscovici suggests that social representations are both conventional and prescriptive. Yet he emphasizes that they are also dynamic, evolving and becoming transformed through communication and interaction. Each individual, he suggests, has a part to play in the way we represent our world (Moscovici 1984b). The essentially fluid nature of social representations makes this theory particularly attractive when studying contemporary societies.

Representations do not just exist in the cognitive sphere, but also in our cultural and historical artefacts. These symbolic representations emerge during social interaction and communication. Joffe (1999) points out that it is refreshing to come across a social psychological theory that makes way for the concept of the 'symbol', so important in other disciplines, and rather underestimated in the social psychological focus on cognition and discourse. She uses the example of the wearing of red ribbons to support AIDS awareness and notes that 'symbols permit people to communicate and to experience a realm beyond the bounds of speech. Meaning is understood without verbal interaction' (1999: 96). When representing death we rely heavily on symbols, such as the use of grey doves in condolence cards, which symbolize the deceased's journey to the afterlife.

Moscovici (1984a) initially claimed that the study of social representations was the study of the dissemination of science, which existed in a 'reified universe', into the 'consensual universe' of collective life via the mass media, thus creating a new 'common sense', made up of a reconstituted 'science'. In effect, Moscovici placed social representations in opposition to science. Purkhardt (1991) notes that this separation of two different types of reality was to prove rather controversial. Our assumption that science is free of the value dimension (Joffe 1999) which is found in mass media is open to question. Fortunately the acceptance that science is itself consensual (Purkhardt 1991) does not detract from the study of the dissemination of scientific ideas into the general population. In this sense, Moscovici's (1976) seminal study of the assimilation of psychoanalytic thought into French society still stands.

Joffe has explored the ways in which knowledge about HIV–AIDS has circulated in populations. It appears that when faced with a terrible new disease both the lay population and scientific communities were active in their efforts to name and to objectify this new phenomenon, as people attempted to understand the origin and spread of the disease. She found that the dominant representations which emerged from this process could be encapsulated by the expression 'not me – others' (1999: 47). The developing representations which were closely associated with the assessment of risk and the attribution of blame drew on ancient cultural themes. For example, in Britain, HIV–AIDS was anchored, by the tabloid press, to the label 'the gay plague'. Joffe found that media representations were loosely based on scientific medical literature, which, significantly, were themselves prone to the exploration and discussion of questionable origin myths that tapped into the theme of blaming out-groups. Joffe argues that the media and government health campaigns acted as important vessels for the dissemination of dominant representations regarding both the origin and the spread of the disease. She suggests that early health campaigns, such as the now-notorious iceberg and tombstone 'advertisements' in Britain, were too fear-evoking, causing a defensive and protective reaction of denial and projection on to the 'other', the 'not me, not my group' reaction (1999: 1).

This realization that science is itself consensual serves to remind us that the presence of science in the Western world does not make contemporary society completely different from those societies without science. The realization that the infiltration of scientific thought does not necessarily cause the collapse of religious and mythical thinking has been dawning on anthropologists for some time. The imagined clean break that contemporary Western society has made with its past is significantly lessened.

Rituals and representations

Moscovici (1984a) has claimed that social representations are an ideal tool for the study of modern, contemporary life where the mass media play a central role. The investigation of this era was to be the task of social psychology. While Moscovici deserves the praise he has gained for adding 'science' to Wundt's (1900–20), list of suitable objects of study (language, religion, customs, myth, magic and cognate phenomena) (Farr 1993), it seems he is also responsible for implicitly excluding myths, custom and ritual in the process. Moscovici appears to view the modern Western world as a land without myths and, as a consequence, a place of empty rituals. In Moscovici's conception of contemporary society, rituals have become profane and habitual. 'Ritual without myth is partial, truncated, [and] does not reach down to the whole being' (Moscovici 1993: 355).

We now come to the question of whether our culture does contain mythical and/or religious thinking. While it would be absurd to suggest that the systems of belief in a complex, heterogeneous, industrial culture would be as coherent or as clear-cut as those found in a tightly knit, organic, non-industrial culture, it is also obvious that religions continue to exist in the former context. Given the intense emotions aroused by death, it is hard to see even the most apparently modern funeral in terms of mere habit. It seems that in his attempt to modernize social representations, Moscovici left behind a key element of culture. In contemporary society, where science and the media play a huge role, rituals and customs are active agents too. This is particularly obvious when we come to study death; the dead cannot just be talked away.

So what is a custom? Or a ritual? Fortunately, when defining ritual we can rely on more than a century's academic wrangling between anthropologists. Seymour-Smith (1986) notes that ritual behaviour is regarded by many anthropologists as a category of behaviour and that a ritual could be defined as a form of ceremony characterized by its religious nature or purpose. Custom presents fewer problems of definition, but is also used less frequently in anthropological text, presumably because customary behaviour is subsumed beneath descriptions of culture. Seymour-Smith provides another useful definition: customs can be seen as cultural traditions or habitual forms of behaviour within a given social group.

Many committal services held in churches or chapels illustrate the features of sacred rituals. In these events, the participants let their minds dwell on the deceased's new start in the afterlife. Such a suspension of rational thought is aided by ritualistic activities such as singing and praying and ritualistic props such as architectural space, incense, altars and clerical robes. The funeral wake, on the other hand, could be described as a mortuary custom. British wakes have a long history and originally preceded the funeral service. Nowadays, people 'wake the dead' after the committal at the local crematorium or cemetery. During a wake the friends and family give a party in honour of the deceased. Typically, sandwiches, cakes and tea or alcohol are served in the house of the deceased, hosted by the closest next of kin.

Collective representations

Moscovici (1984a) identified Durkheim, a powerful force in both sociology and anthropology (Lukes 1973), as the ancestor of the theory. This clearly marked out his theory as belonging to a sociological tradition of research and went some way in helping him achieve his goal of forging closer links with the social disciplines of anthropology and history (Moscovici 1984b). Yet Deutscher (1984: 98) argues that Moscovici has only used one of Durkheim's ideas in isolation – that of the representation – and that he should not feel obligated to identify Durkheim as the ancestor. Deutscher is not alone in his reservations concerning the choice of just Durkheim as the ancestor of the theory (Farr 1987).

In 1898 Durkheim distinguished collective representations from individual representations. Durkheim argued that while sociologists should study collective representations, the study of individual representations was the domain of psychologists (Farr 1998). Farr notes that these collective representations had a great deal in common with Wundt's *Völkerpsychologie* (1900–20). Durkheim, who had been impressed by Wundt's psychological laboratory when he visited it had, apparently, more mixed feelings about Wundt's proposal that collective phenomena could also be studied as a part of psychology (Giddens 1978). Durkheim's distinction between collective and individual representations forced a split between sociology and psychology. The individualist psychology that Durkheim was rejecting became the dominant form of both psychology and social psychology (Farr 1998) and thus Durkheim 'created an identity crisis for social psychologists which they have been unable to resolve in the course of the twentieth century'(1998: 277).

Yet sociological forms of social psychology have developed. Farr (1998) argues that when Moscovici, in his attempt to 'modernize' social representations (1984b), renamed this 'neglected concept of Durkheim's' (Moscovici 1976) 'social' rather than 'collective' he was as keen as Durkheim had been to distinguish his social representations from a conception of individual representations that would operate like attitudes or opinions, to be found isolated within individuals. Moscovici's social representations were envisioned as being 'more dynamic, continually changing and less widely shared than ever before' (Farr 1998: 285). These social representations of science made 'common', which were circulated by the mass media, seemed different from the kind of collective representation found in premodern societies.

To a large degree, Moscovici's attempt at modernization was successful. The social representation appears to work. However, Farr argues that there is a dominant 'collective' representation in the West which, by its very character, blinds us to the fact that it permeates society. He argues that the collective representation of the individual 'is a representation that individualises other collective representations' (Farr 1998: 286). Thus individualism, identified as a force in modernity (Lukes 1973), can be viewed as a collective representation 'in the full Durkheimian sense of the term' (Farr 1996: 104). So while Farr acknowledges that individualism can be a by-product of social change, he also suggests that individualism can operate as a 'social fact' (Farr 1998: 287). For example, the collective representation of the individual's responsibility for their actions lies at the very heart of the social representations of the 'good' or 'bad' death and the 'healthy' or 'unhealthy' grief reactions described in this book. Seen in these terms we can understand why using 'individualism' as the organizing concept to explain developments in our mortuary practices and representations of death may not be particularly fruitful.

It is possible that we are about to enter into an era of collective representations. Farr (1998) suggests that in these times of globalization there may be a place for this concept. Interestingly, Jahoda's (1988: 196) assertion that the notion of collective representations is 'valuable for anthropologists concerned with small-scale homogeneous cultures' may also apply to the social scientist exploring aspects of culture in the global village of the twenty-first century.

Summary and conclusion

In this chapter I have sought to find a way of understanding contemporary British death practices from a social psychological perspective. In order to avoid the pitfall of placing findings in an atheoretical sub-specialism called 'the social psychology of death' (see Mellor 1993; Bauman 1992a), I am making use of the theory of social representations, established by Moscovici, and the work of Mead and of Goffman. My study therefore lies in a social tradition of research founded on the philosophy of Hegel. Naturally, adopting this Hegelian position will enable me to make use of both anthropology and sociology. In the chapters that follow, I explore the role played by contemporary death customs and rituals in the production and reproduction of representations of death.

Our deathways exist in time and place and I have attempted to give a brief social history of British death practices. Death practices have been undergoing relatively rapid transformations for almost 150 years and the period while I was in the field was no exception. I saw the launch of the natural death movement, discussed in some detail in Chapter 6. I also attended a cemetery and crematoria conference in which I learned about the proposal for the rapid exhumations of buried corpses as a means to overcome the full cemeteries surrounding our urban centres and of the proposal to start up new 'green' cemeteries, in which headstones were to be replaced by trees.

2 Researching death
An urban ethnography

The choice of qualitative methodologies

The cultural strategies, metaphors and taboos that characterize humanity's responses to death can best be accessed through qualitative methodologies. This is a topic in which every action appears to be invested with layers of meaning and it is particularly helpful to adopt an open-ended approach. Not knowing in advance what conclusions will be drawn from the research project is a positive feature of qualitative studies. However, being 'open-ended' or flexible in our approach is very different from being without structure or unable to ground the data in theory. In the simultaneous process of data collection and analysis I used the theory of social representations, described in the previous chapter.

I have taken my inspiration from field studies by Humpheys (1970), Festinger *et al.* (1956) and Hockey (1990), among others. These authors acknowledge their own salience as participants in both the 'field' and the text. As I shall illustrate in this chapter, my presence during the fieldwork had an effect on what people did or said. Further, my life experience and personality has had an incalculable impact not only on the interpretations I made of the data, but also on the way in which I present this material in written form. As Hockey points out in her introduction to her fieldwork in a nursing home, her research did not so much as unearth data 'out there' as create findings which were 'the outcome of a protracted, intersubjective process' (Hockey 1990: 6).

Such an approach represents something of a departure from traditional social psychological research in which quantitative methodologies dominate. With the exception of social psychologists such as Radley (1993, 1994), who argues for the use of qualitative research methods, most social psychological studies are positivistic. Keen to align itself to the natural sciences and interested in the study of small groups of individuals, this discipline has always been more at home with quantitative research methods rather than the more 'woolly' data-collection procedures characterized by the long in-depth interview or the participant observation study in the field.

Despite the fact that social representations are best accessed through qualitative methodologies, even a review of English-speaking social representations' literature produces few truly qualitative studies. The use of inappropriate quantitative methodologies suggests that for many, including Moscovici, the transition to a sociological form of social psychology has not been easy. In 1985 Semin argued that 'much of the research employing the "notion" of social representations does not amount to an alternative to the dominant mode of social psychology, either conceptually or empirically' (cf. Abric 1984; Codol 1984; Flament 1984) (Semin 1985: 93). The preference for quantitative studies also helps to explain why there has been so little research into the role of customs and rituals which cannot be sensibly explored by quantitative research techniques.

Joffe (1999) identifies two strands of research in the field. In one, the 'social' is defined as the sharing of attitudes; thus in order to access these shared representations we merely have to survey, using quantitative methodologies, opinions 'out there' in society. But as Joffe points out, people may respond to a social representation and yet not be consciously aware that they are doing so. Access to such representations is not possible through efforts of tapping consensuality, she argues. The second strand of research seeks to find an understanding of social representations 'both as **environment** and as entities that exist in people's minds' (Joffe 1999: 98, original emphasis). Therefore to understand social representations we have to look at culture as well as at what people have to say. Access to such information is available through a process of triangulation in which several methodologies, such as the analysis of texts from the media, participant observation and interviewing, are used to gain an understanding of the 'genesis, circulation and transformation of knowledge in a society, as well as the workings of dominant thinking' (Joffe 1999: 99).

In a theory that focuses on the circulation of knowledge, as expressed in cultural artefacts, talk and behaviour, the striking avoidance of qualitative research methodologies has been a disappointment. However, exemplary exceptions to this trend are provided by Jodelet (1991), who looked at social representations of madness in a French community, Chombart de Lauwe (1984), who explored representations of childhood and Joffe's (1999) analysis of the social representations of risk.

The role of pilot work

Any piece of social research benefits greatly from a period of free-ranging, open-minded exploration. This is called pilot work. There is nothing mysterious about undertaking pilot work. Pilot work is based on common sense; in a nutshell, the researcher goes out and visits people and places, they interview people and listen in on conversations, they take notes, go home, write a few 'memos' (these can be filed under various headings, such as 'methodology', 'theory', etc.), they have a think and, finally, construct a few research questions. In my study, I listed all those institutions which 'dealt' with death, such as hospices, hospitals, registry offices, coroners' offices, funeral parlours, crematoria and cemeteries. Having drawn up this list I then set out to visit these 'death sites'. I then formulated a second list of people who work in these institutions. I began to hold informal chats with funeral directors; I sat in on bereavement support groups, interviewed therapists and bereavement counsellors; I talked to attendants at crematoria and cemetery managers. This was a period of intense 'memoing' and note-taking as I attempted to build up some kind of picture of contemporary, urban British death practices.

The 'first days in the field' can be confusing and tough. I well remember spending long days in unfamiliar places, asking inappropriate questions. I suffered agonies of self-consciousness and self-doubt that were made all the more acute given the emotional and sensitive nature of the topic. Researching death in our own culture can be uncomfortable. However, a thorough pilot study is worthwhile and can alter the whole direction of the final main study. That was the case in the present project.

Primed by my reading in psychopathology which included analyses of pathological grief reactions, I began my research with an interest in the 'grief outcomes' of the bereaved next of kin. I launched into a few pilot interviews with women who had lost their husbands some months previously. Fortunately, rather than set my own agenda by presenting the 'subject' with a questionnaire or list of research questions about grief, I held relatively free-ranging interviews. Although their descriptions of sorrow were all too lucid, I soon found that their accounts were not dominated by talk about insomnia or an inability to concentrate on things, but by the social experience of bereavement. For example, the women talked in great depth about the days leading up to the death; they vividly described the moment of death; they articulated their views on medical care; they talked about their relationship with the funeral director; they shared their thoughts on embalming; they told me about their fights with bureaucrats regarding insurance or social security claims and they often told me about their altered status as a widow. I found these descriptive passages peopled by family, friends, work colleagues, pets and dozens of deathwork professionals. The accounts of loss were tainted by medical, commercial and bureaucratic concerns. Reformulating my research questions, I began to move away from an exploration of grief symptoms and focused instead on the cultural organization, or constructions, of dying, death and bereavement.

The main study

Generally, pilot studies have a natural 'shelf life'. After a while, we find we are able to anticipate the general topics and broad themes that will emerge from a day in the field. This kind of saturation does not tend to occur so quickly in a main study, because the fine-tuned research questions generate their own data and make the data-collection process more complex and interesting. The researcher undertaking a pilot study is more like a journalist than a social scientist – they do make discoveries, but they are really just skimming the surface. After three or four months of pilot work I had reached a stage where I could articulate my new research questions, some of which are described below. As I was undertaking a qualitative research project, I was aware that these research questions were not fixed. I would need to restate my hypotheses having considered the in-coming data.

I had by now developed an interest in the cultural constructions of death. By this I mean I was keen to unravel the meaning behind the apparently normal acts which constitute our social organization of death: why do funeral directors move bodies from the hospital mortuary in unmarked vans? Why are men, rather than women, seen as more able to cope with the sight of a disfigured corpse? Why do we spend so much time and money embalming a corpse that is cremated two days later? What do we mean when we say someone had a 'good death'? What happens when there is no body? From these vague and apparently disparate questions I began to distil my central research hypotheses.

Influenced by the work of the anthropologists Durkheim (1915), Hertz (1960) and Van Gennup (1960) I began to conceptualize contemporary British deaths as representing some kind of threat to the existing social order. I imagined that the survivors responded to the threat of disorder by participating in a variety of death customs and rituals. Yet in this industrialized, urbanized and multicultural society I could not expect the pattern of responses to be necessarily coherent. Drawing on the work of the anthropologist Douglas (1966, 1973), I was interested in looking at the way in which we react to the dead body. Faced by the shocking and inert corpse, I was intrigued to observe our reactions to an object that has the appearance of humanity yet lacks its essence. What we do to the corpse may not necessarily be so rational or scientific, but symbolic, representing a discourse about death, an analysis of which provides insights not only into our views of mortality, but also into the very social fabric of contemporary culture. By this I mean a glimpse into the distribution of the social order, control and power. Our reaction to death is made more complex by the relatively recent handing over of the process of dying and the acts of disposal to groups of specially trained deathwork professionals. Making use of the sociologist Goffman (1959), I wanted to look at the ways in which our death practices are dramatized between deathwork professional and grieving client. Finally, making use of the social psychological theory championed by Moscovici (1984a) I wanted to explore how representations of death and loss both shape and are shaped by our mortuary practices. For example, what is the nature of the interplay between a representation of the good death and the practice of embalming? These became my working hypotheses which were shaped by and in turn shaped my fieldwork.

Participating and observing

Participant observation lends itself to certain research environments. Particularly suitable are those situations in which the researcher wishes to know more about unusual or idiosyncratic 'small worlds'. Certainly, the 'small world' of the deathwork professional would seem to fit the description. Funeral directors and crematorium attendants run most of their operations behind the scenes, hidden from view. For example, very few people know what an embalmer does when they embalm a body. We are unlikely to know what tools they may use. We may not have ever paused to consider what qualifications they have acquired and we are most unlikely to be familiar with the appearance of an embalming room. Knowledge about the funeral industry is not general knowledge. Until quite recently, detailed information about the social organization of death in contemporary

Britain was scanty even within the academic world. For example, Howarth's taboo-breaking ethnographic account of funeral-directing was published in 1996. Research into this field requires familiarity with sites, scenes, conversations and behaviour which at first may seem extraordinary. Participant observation provides the ideal means to such an end (Jorgensen 1989).

> By participant observation we mean that method in which the observer participates in the daily life of the people under study, either openly or in the role of researcher or covertly in some disguised role, observing things that happen, listening to what is said, and questioning people, over some length of time.
>
> (Becker and Geer 1969: 322)

McCall and Simmons' (1969) definition of participant observation is very useful: indeed, it describes my fieldwork. They suggest that it should involve some genuine social interaction in the field, direct observation of relevant events, some formal and informal interviewing, some systematic counting, some collection of documents—artefacts and an open mind in regard to the direction that the study might take. For a fuller description of the practice of participant observation I would direct the reader to the works of Becker (1958), Lofland (1971) and Burgess (1984, 1985) and Malinowski (1922).

A major difficulty facing the budding participant observer is the issue of gaining access. Jorgensen (1989) outlines two distinct entry strategies: overt and covert. Overt approaches entail gaining permission from those in power through formal applications. We can then allow personal contacts to 'snowball' at both upper and lower levels of an institution's hierarchical structure. Naturally, this sort of overt approach is necessary if we wish to enter into any kind of participatory role. Covert entry strategies, associated with straight observation, spare us from negotiation; we simply arrive at the site in question and set to work 'mingling'. Most of my fieldwork 'entries' were overt. Indeed, I wrote so many letters to funeral parlours, hospitals, crematoria, etc. at the beginning of my fieldwork that I felt more like a secretary than a social scientist. Ideally, we would hire someone else to do this job to avoid the problem of the researcher entering the fieldwork situation feeling indebted to the very people they are about to 'study'.

People are naturally wary of psychologists and, in my experience, slightly alarmed by qualitative researchers who are not clutching a questionnaire booklet. The psychologist in the field may have to rely on their persuasive powers. As Johnson (1976) rather sourly notes, it is perhaps worth appreciating that 'gaining entry' is not so much about being 'nice' and 'honest', but about being cunning, deceptive and using whatever power we have. To gain entry from people in authority we have to present an artificially concise 'cover story' when, in reality, we know full well that we will not know what form or character the research findings will take for many months. Finally, however clearly we try to explain what happens during the research process, we can discover that those who have agreed to take part in a study imagined something very different. A funeral director, having agreed to let me 'observe the day-to-day activities of his firm', absolutely refused to let me see his workshop or any backstage areas of his parlour; for him, research meant interviewing. In such instances, I had little choice but to adapt to the restraints of the situation. I never did get to see his embalming room.

It is useful to remember the issue of motivation. Wax (1952), working on a model of reciprocity, identifies the following, somewhat depressing, reasons why people agree to help in social research: lone-liness, boredom, curiosity, ego and vanity. In similar vein, Agar (1980), discussing cross-cultural ethnographies, warns of the dangers of the researcher becoming involved with 'stranger-handlers'. These individuals may be outsiders and may be more likely to approach a social scientist than those who are highly integrated into the community in question. While we might not expect marginalized 'stranger-handlers' to be such an issue in a same-culture study (I am presuming it is easier to identify the marginalized in our own culture), I found it was useful to ascertain the status of those who appeared too willing or over-keen to take part in research; sometimes they did not make the best informants. Meanwhile, the researcher should remain aware of their motivations. For example, there is a real danger that the researcher will seek out those who are articulate, educated and who 'speak their language', thus introducing an element of bias (Campbell 1969). This is particularly tempting when carrying out same-culture studies.

> Any group of persons – prisoners, primitives, pilots, or patients – develop a life of their own that becomes meaningful, reasonable, and normal once you get close to it, and that a good way to learn about any of these worlds is to submit oneself in the company of the members to the daily round of petty contingencies to which they are subject.
>
> (Goffman: preface to *Asylums* 1961)

The organization of death in contemporary Britain takes place in many locations: the hospital, the register office, the coroner's office, the funeral parlour, the crematorium and the cemetery. Staff members within these very different institutions or sites are loosely held together by their common activity and their mutual aims: namely to discover, report and note the cause of a death and to dispose of a corpse. The deathwork professional would appear to represent an example of Harré's 'structured group', i.e. a group of individuals who are bound together by 'rights, obligations and duties that yield characteristic kinds of action from each role-holder' (Harré 1984: 932).

At first the extent and form of my sample was chosen on the basis of my pilot study. I was aware of certain formal categories of organization and interviewed at least one person from each category, although I usually interviewed more (a hospital chaplain, a parish priest, hospital nurses from different types of wards, a patients' affairs officer, a registrar, police officers from various divisions, a coroner, etc.). However, during the main study I developed an increased understanding of the situation and environment and began to undertake 'theoretical sampling' (Strauss 1987). By this I mean I purposely chose subjects to compare with those spoken to previously. For example, having spoken to several traditional family-run funeral directors, I sought out an interview with a business involved in aggressive buy-outs of old family-run firms. This enabled me to compare the widely differing perspectives and aspirations of the old and the new. This kind of sampling decision was very much conditioned by my frame of reference but, as Zelditch (1969) notes, this is acceptable.

By its nature, a participant observation study offers the researcher various sources of data. These come in many different forms. One source comes from the informants' knowledge, which can be gleaned from casual conversation or in-depth, unstructured and structured interviews. We can also use documents, audio-recorders, photographs, video-recorders, artefacts and a personal fieldwork diary or log. I chose not to make a video diary of my fieldwork; at the time the idea of videoing other people's funerals did not feel right. I made use of all the other sources of data, such as audio-recorders, etc. Because the primary method of data collection in participant observation is direct observation, it is worth remembering that much 'data' exists as the experience and acquired knowledge of the researcher.

Choosing the right kind of role for the researcher is very important. Geer (1969) suggests that fieldworkers should try not to stand out as different from those whom they are studying. We should be neutral, yet approachable. Maintaining such a role can be a strain and, of course, much depends on the topic under study. For example, in their classic study of a Messianic cult, Festinger *et al.* (1956), posing as new converts, tried to adopt a bland and non-committal stance. As it turned out, this middle-of-the-road mildness aroused great suspicion from fellow cult members who were, after all, anticipating the end of the world. Similarly, when researching death, we have to get the balance right between the quest for good data and the need to adapt to social situations which are often emotional. I had to live with myself after a day in the field; I was cautious.

Degrees of participation over observation can vary from study to study, ranging from full participation to full observation. Rose (1982) has identified the following sets of fieldwork roles: complete participation; participant-as-observer; observer-as-participant; and complete observer. Another way of looking at these various roles is to think of them as insider versus outsider. The full participant has become an 'insider', the complete observer remains an 'outsider'. As Hockey (1990) notes, it should not be the researcher's goal to become totally immersed in the field as we then lose the ability to self-consciously analyse the situation. Thus, the role adopted has a great impact on incoming data. During the data-collection process and the analysis and presentation of the data it is important to keep in mind which roles were used and to think about what influence this may have had on things.

So what kind of balance between participant–observer or insider–outsider did I achieve in my roles as researcher? Researching the social organization of death requires that we follow the corpse from site to site, institution to institution. In such a multisite study I was always on the move and it was not feasible to aim for a 'complete participant', insider, role. Mainly, I adopted the role of observer-as-participant. I carried out a series of trips to various 'death sites' such as hospitals, mortuary chapels, coroner's courts, murder investigation rooms at police stations, funeral parlours, etc. More interactive and involved than a passive observer, I would interview, converse and even lend a helping hand if it seemed appropriate (which was rare). Gold (1969) has suggested that such research relationships are superficial and he argues that we run serious risks of misunderstanding the informant's statements. He has a point. Sadly, without an unlimited time scale or an endless budget, observer-as-participant research roles are the most sensible option available to the social scientist who wishes to understand multisite phenomena.

Sometimes I found it useful to adopt the role of complete observer.

On such occasions, I would visit public places, such as crematoria or cemeteries, and observe the day's comings and goings. The visiting general public and many of the members of staff were unaware of the presence of a watching social scientist. Spared from direct social interaction, we lose the perspective of the participants but gain the advantage of an opportunity for more objective observation. Adopting such a role can make us feel uncomfortable as we cannot hide behind the (illusionary) distance of cross-cultural research or the comforting safety of 'informed consent'.

Of course, we cannot observe or participate in everything – certain phenomena occur too erratically or maybe are taboo or private. In such instances we need to turn to informants. Indeed, Agar (1980) suggests that recorded interviews with key informants should be viewed as the primary source of data, with observation holding a supplementary, though important, role. These long interviews, which often spanned several hours, provided the bulk of my participant observation data. As Howarth (1993) has observed, informants are usually pleased to be given the opportunity to 'tell it like it is'. I found this to be the case and I rarely had to use prompts. On the other hand, while it is important to leave these interviews relatively unstructured, so that we do not impose our world view on the informant, it is also useful to have some idea about where the interview will go. I kept an interview guide, which outlined my developing interests and concepts, which I would consult either if things began to flag or if I felt that the interview was going a bit 'wild'. Now while the questions I asked in such instances were without doubt 'leading', this was not neces- sarily a bad thing. All questions are, by their nature, leading. Indeed, Agar (1980) has suggested that we sometimes need to 'bully' the respondents in order to pursue a topic that they may prefer to avoid. Common sense and tact must be used in the deployment of such a strategy. In the sample of script given below I was asking a casualty doctor who was working in a busy London hospital about breaking bad news after a death.

MB: 'How long do you yourself spend with relatives?
Doctor: 'Myself?'
MB: 'Honestly'
Doctor: 'Er, five minutes?'

There are times when the researcher has to ask questions about the answers, too. We may be unsure whether we have understood what the informant means and this cannot be achieved by simply parroting back the words of the subject. My self-reflective informants also wanted to check on my meanings or understanding. The ability to negotiate is an essential tool in this research process.

Dean and Whyte (1969), in a chapter ominously entitled *How do you know if the informant is telling the truth?* have addressed the issue of the veracity of informants' statements. They stress the importance of distinguishing between statements that are clearly objective, such as 'I am a funeral director', and those that are subjective, 'and my fees are very reasonable'. They warn the researcher to be aware of ulterior motives, bars to spontaneity, the desire to please and various unspeci-fied idiosyncratic factors. Fortunately, they offer the reader some checks to plausibility, such as the inherent implausibility of the tale, the unreliability of the informant, knowledge about the inform-ant's mental set and the comparison of informants' accounts with other forms of data.

A multisite study could be characterized as a series of meetings and partings. I regularly found myself in the position of 'leaving the field'. Given the more superficial nature of the research relationship, saying goodbye to an informant is not as significant as it would be after many months of research in one site in close company with a few subjects, yet, in my experience, leaving the field can still be an odd moment. While the fieldworker may feel somewhat relieved, already thinking of their next fieldwork site, the research informant may feel rather insecure. 'I haven't stopped talking,' exclaimed a member of the CID who had been describing murder investigations. 'That's the problem, I think I'd better take a copy of that tape!' He did not, but his comment illustrates the unease that can be caused by taking part in social research. To lessen my respondent's apprehension I always tried to end the exchange with some kind of debriefing session, although this was not always possible. In these I would discuss what had been covered in the interview. I would also restate the research project's aims and describe what form the final product would take. Finally, I would repeat my promises to maintain the respondent's anonymity and to respect their confidentiality.

'Inter-viewing'

To a certain extent my interviews with bereaved women could be viewed as an extension of my participant observation key informant interviews. However, I have decided to describe these under a separate heading as there were certain differences in the way in which I chose subjects and the ways in which I conducted the interviews. Most importantly, these interviews were very different because I was not talking to deathwork professionals, for whom death was safely abstracted, but to people who had lost someone they loved. The twelve women who spoke to me told me stories of loss that were intimate, touching, even humorous at times. Most of all they were always, always heart-breaking.

Interviews are such a common event in our daily lives that it is easy to overlook the subtle processes that are at work whenever two or more people share information through talk. In 1982 Farr provided the theoretical framework for interviewing which was first called for by Cannell and Kahn back in 1968. Rather than merely providing another guide on how to conduct interviews (for example, Douglas 1985), Farr attempts to unravel the internal dynamics of the interview. In order to emphasize the interactive two-way process that is at the heart of this form of social exchange and in order to draw our attention to the fact that most interviews make use of both auditory and visual channels of communication, Farr prefers to call the interview the 'inter-view'.

> An inter-view is a social encounter between two or more individuals with words as the main medium of exchange. It is, in short, a peculiar form of conversation in which the ritual of turn-taking is more formalised than in the commoner and more informal encounters of everyday life.
>
> (Farr 1982: 151)

Drawing on Heider's (1958) distinction between the perceiver, 'P', and the other, 'O', Goffmann's (1959) dramaturgical observations concerning the performances of daily life and Mead's (1934) belief that the meaning of an act is to be found in the response that it elicits from observing others, Farr developed a social psychology of the interview. At the core of this theory, he was keen to emphasize the co-existence of more than one perspective. During an interview both the interviewee and the interviewer, who may well swap roles, negotiate around a quite natural divergence of perspectives. Seen in these terms traditional concepts of interview 'bias' can be reinterpreted as an intrinsic part of the exchange; so rather than viewing the researcher as 'contaminating' the interview data, it is more useful to understand the researcher as a vital participant in the production of that data – no researcher, no subject, no inter-view. Farr's view of the interview has much in common with anthropological and sociological descriptions of participation observation.

I took a practical decision to interview widows. Statistically women live longer than men, so there are more widows to interview. Constrained by time and person-power it was simply easier to get access to the larger pool of bereaved women. Further, as I wished to interview people in their homes, I felt it was prudent to stick to my own gender. There were advantages to be gained from this decision. Oakley found that her female respondents made assumptions about her shared experience, causing her to abandon traditional, 'masculine' guidelines of objectivity in an interview (Oakley 1993). Certainly I found that my intimate interviews with bereaved women did not conform to any idealized image of a formal exchange (see Radley 1994).

However, I am well aware that, by focusing on female conjugal bereavement, I am continuing a tradition of research that excludes not only widowers but the surviving partners of other couples, such as gay, extra-marital or non-married relationships. The intensity of grief could be the same for any of these groups of bereaved people, although the social experience of loss, in certain instances, may be skewed by the public's failure to perceive who really are the 'primary bereaved'. During my fieldwork I was told the story of a woman who was denied access to her lover's body in the hospital mortuary because his wife had already been to view him. Central in the deceased's life while he was alive, this woman found herself painfully marginalized once he was dead. Finally, it is worth remembering that there are many other kinds of dyadic relationships, such as parent–child, friend, sibling and colleague, all of which can be torn apart by death and any of which would make worthy material for research. Raphael (1984) provides an excellent account of these various types of bereavement and the repercussions of such loss.

Finding people willing to talk about their bereavement was not easy. This is a group of people who deserve protection. I had to rely on volunteers and I made up my small sample through requests in the national press, through the help of the bereavement-support group Cruse and a funeral director who had a parlour in London. The women I interviewed came from a wide range of socioeconomic backgrounds and ages. Choosing an appropriate timespan after the death in which to interview this highly vulnerable sample was difficult. In the end I chose to interview respondents seven to eleven months after their bereavement. This gave them time to make some small progress in coming to terms with their loss. I avoided interviewing people at the time of the first, painful anniversary of the death (Bornstein *et al.* 1973; Carey 1977, 1979; Pollock 1970).

Although we are a culture that is familiar with social research and commercial surveys, taking part in bereavement research shortly after a death does represent a departure from the social norm. I am not sure how I would respond to a request to be interviewed after the death of my partner. It is therefore worthwhile to look at the issue of respondent motivation. At the end of the long interviews I asked the women why they had agreed to take part in the study. Their reasons were varied. Several women discussed the need for more studies to be carried out in this field and said that they were keen to help in research. One woman was very angry about the bad treatment she had had from a funeral director and she said she wanted to complain to someone. Two respondents had been encouraged to take part by other family members who perhaps had in mind some idea of a therapeutic interview. One woman admitted that she needed to talk to someone, anyone, even me. Another woman had not had a guest in her home for three months and I guessed that loneliness was also her motive.

Whatever these women's motivation, I remain grateful to them for letting me into their homes at such a time. I shall never forget these interviews. Presented with a young interviewer, the women responded with accounts of their husband's death that were frank, honest and profound. They had not only lost their partner: over the span of a few months many aspects of their lifestyle, identity and status had also changed. Most of the women were struggling to come to terms with their new role as a single person. They were often short of money, nearly always suffered from loneliness and were, to a woman, full of sorrow. On some occasions surrounded by a sea of cakes and sandwiches, I would listen to their stories of love and loss. I was often near tears. Death concentrates the mind and people who have watched someone they love die do a great deal of thinking. Certainly many of the women impressed me with their wisdom and maturity.

The experience of being interviewed is all too familiar to a bereaved person who, having arranged a funeral, has become used to these formal conversations with professionals. Further, in our culture we are constantly bombarded with interviews on radio and television. The media teach us how to take part in interviews. So perhaps it is not surprising that I found my respondents relatively confident at the start of the interviews. I had expected them to be more intimidated by the recorder than they appeared to be. One woman asked to have a copy of the tape, which I sent her. I understood that she wanted to give it to her son, as she had felt that she had not been able to communicate with him face to face.

Our culture is often ambivalent about women without men. Indeed, at the time I was conducting my research Scottish Widows was airing a series of televised advertisements in which a young woman stalked around a set in a black hooded cape. I was not without certain fears. Unfamiliar with death, I superstitiously worried that I would in some way be contaminated by the bereavements I was hearing about. I soon came to realize that these women were 'normal'. People often express their sense of embarrassment when faced with the newly bereaved. What does one say? I have to admit that it was sometimes a relief to hide behind my research role which required me to listen, not talk.

So during the interviews I did not say very much. On the basis of the pilot study, I had settled on the following opening question: 'I would like you to talk about all you remember of the few days prior to your husband's death, the day he died, and the week or so that followed'. The respondents would then launch into their story, usually approaching it chronologically. Most of my communication was non-verbal consisting of head-nods, smiles and such like. Although I had extensive 'probe questions' ready to hand, I rarely had to use them. This first half of the interview could take several hours and could be harrowing. The women often broke down as they remembered some poignant detail. When this happened I would switch off the recorder and would either quietly wait in silence or, if it seemed appropriate, I would say how helpful she was being and how privileged I was to hear what she had to say. When the woman felt she could continue we would start up the tape again. Ann and Christine (not their real names) cried so much and so often that in the end we just kept on recording. Talking about death cannot always be a dry subject.

After a break we would enter the second phase of the interview in which I asked some questions about various aspects of the experience of being bereaved. For example, I asked them whether they felt they had been prepared for their husband's death and how they would describe the death. I explored other issues, too, such as their sense of satisfaction (or otherwise) with the funeral arrangements and what improvements they thought could be made to our death system.

I was aware that an upsetting interview could be hard on the women and I felt it was particularly important to carry out some kind of debriefing exercise in these interviews. A morning spent talking about the death and bereavement was clearly going to revive the pain of the loss. In the third stage of the interview I attempted to wind things down by lightening the tone. I asked the women what advice they would give to a newly bereaved person. This was a popular question as it allowed the women to be active, practical and helpful. While the advice they offered drew a painful picture of loss (for example, 'eat with the radio on, it makes you feel less lonely'), on more than one occasion the women surprised me by their humorous warnings about amorous widowers, roving husbands and jealous wives. At this stage the conversation would often move on to other topics. For example, I would be shown family snapshots and other memorabilia. While I tried to create a reasonably cheerful atmosphere, I have no doubt that the women were exhausted after I had gone.

The data

Various types of data were produced by the participant-observation study and the in-depth interviews with the women. In both halves of the study I ended up with 'field notes' which are by their very nature, subjective. It is important to be sensitive about writing out these notes while in the field, for there is nothing more off-putting than a jotting social scientist. I would usually make these notes on my way home or later on in the day. I noted the obvious, concrete details such as the who, what, when and where of the research. I also included more impressionistic, judgemental and apparently trivial material, such as what people wore, whether food or drink was offered, observations on the participants' apparent state of mind. I also wrote about my feelings and the emotions aroused by the exchange. These were often complex. It took a certain amount of defence to stride into the world of death and bereavement. If I quoted statements made by subjects, I was careful to distinguish between my own speech and that of my respondents.

Another source of data took the form of documents. As Zelditch has noted (1969) these are usually unsystematically obtained. This was certainly true in my own experience. I collected various forms connected with the organization of the funeral, such as the cremation forms. I picked up application forms for 'Pay now, die later' funerals. I collected a fascinating sample of trade brochures advertising cremators, ashes urns and a whole selection of memorial artefacts. It was rare for me to come away from a day's fieldwork empty-handed.

From both sets of ethnographic interviews I ended up with two important artefacts: the interview tapes themselves and, later, the transcriptions. I transcribed many hours of recorded interviews. This was an arduous task that took more than three months. Listening and relistening to the same chunks of speech certainly made me very familiar with the data. During this time I became embedded in talk about death. I made many memos while I transcribed. These were simply thoughts, ideas or hunches concerning my research. Sometimes I wrote a few lines; other times I took several pages of notes. These dated and titled memos were periodically resorted and labelled under various broad headings, such as 'ritual', 'commercial concerns', 'theory', 'methodology', etc. The memos form the groundwork for the analysis that follows.

Although I have dedicated a separate section to the topic of data analysis, which can be found in the Appendix, I must emphasize that the process of data analyses went hand-in-hand with the procedures of data collection. Moving from straight descriptive observation, in which I asked myself a series of questions concerning context and behaviour in each site and situation, I could begin to make more focused observations, in which I compared and contrasted and in which I actively sought out discrepancies. Hypotheses were formulated on the basis of this incoming data and these were verified against further data.

> [Field research] promises a theoretical understanding of socially meaningful activities as experienced by the members of society, at least in so far as this is possible. It promises an understanding grounded in the realities of daily life rather than one which reflects the observer's perceptual faith or the realities of an academic subculture.
>
> (Johnson 1976: 211)

Ethical considerations

Earlier I mentioned one of the ethical dilemmas facing a social scientist researching death: that of gaining access. Precisely at a time when respondents want to know exactly what the study is about, the researcher is in a state of open-minded free-enquiry. In order to achieve that much coveted access it is necessary to present a digestible 'cover-story' about the research aims. I suspect I would not have got very far had I said 'I want to examine the interactions between the deathwork professional and the bereaved client. Although I am not sure what I will find at the moment, I want to look at our current social representations of death.' Instead, I would settle with saying that I was studying 'the funeral industry', or 'attitudes towards death', or 'looking at the experience of arranging the funeral'. As you can see, my cover-story was somewhat flexible.

The biggest ethical dilemma I had to face was the issue of approaching bereaved people and asking them to volunteer to take part in research interviews. Ethical committees are becoming very cautious about giving researchers access to such vulnerable individuals as these. People who have just suffered a bereavement should be protected, but it is also important that we do not blindly follow cultural restrictions that merely express our discomfort with the topic of death. The sentiments, views and opinions of people facing this universal experience need to be heard if we are to forge a humanistic response to death and bereavement. In all exchanges I made every effort to be sensitive. However, I was often painfully aware that the interviews sometimes caused distress. Talking about loss and death is rarely easy.

Throughout my research I made attempts to respect my respondents' anonymity and confidentiality. On the day after collecting the data, pseudonyms replaced real names and I continued this practice throughout the research process. I was careful not to reveal to anyone the names of those businesses or institutions that took part in the study. Given that some of the material I collected could be considered controversial, I made the decision to keep the raw data out of the public sphere. To this day I am the only person who has listened to the tapes or read the full transcripts. When quotations or descriptions do occur in the book, the identities of the people and places described in the book are heavily disguised. So while my respondents may recognize their feelings and points of view, I trust they will not see themselves on the printed page.

Hockey (1990) discusses the way in which her gender and age influenced her treatment as a fieldworker in nursing homes. She notes that she was pigeon-holed by staff as a nice middle-class mum. Caring about the elderly was a natural extension of her role as housewife and mother. In such a role she enjoyed the advantages of getting backstage. The reaction may have been very different had she been a male academic. I certainly found that my status as a young married woman worked for me in the fieldwork situation. Women are very often perceived as being good listeners and I made the most of this. My age and gender did not always work for me, however. Although the women I spoke to came from a range of age groups from mid-thirties to mid-seventies, I was the same age as some of the women's daughters and this undoubtedly influenced their reactions to me. I interviewed one particular woman who had two daughters my age who tried to spare me the painful details. She was very clear that this was her aim for her offspring but it was only months later when I was analysing the text of the interview that I was struck by the motherly tone of her account.

I noticed that I was often 'familiarized' in the in-depth interviews with the grieving women by being anchored in the role of counsellor. My letters of reference came from a department of social psychology. This had an impact that I had not anticipated. 'Social psychology' was sometimes interpreted as 'therapy'. Several times during the interviews I found myself being asked for my 'professional' opinion on matters. Alternatively, I was informed that I was being confided in. At times, this seemed like a weighty responsibility. I always found the assumption that I could in some way help very disconcerting as I did not see my interviews in therapeutic terms. If anything, they seemed to be quite the reverse.

In contrast to this familiarization of the researcher as counsellor, during my participant observation I was more often likened to some kind of journalist: a sort of academic private detective. Unusual facts, juicy details, suggestions for further research through contacts or sites and other such titbits were given to me with great enthusiasm. Howarth (1993: 230), in an account of investigating deathwork in funeral parlours, which involved sitting in on arrangement interviews, mentions how we may become embroiled in mild deceits. For example, neatly dressed in black skirt and white blouse, as instructed by her host, she found that the funeral director would implicitly present her to the grieving relatives as a trainee undertaker. I had much the same experience in a funeral-directing firm. By some alchemy which did not involve anyone saying anything, I found myself being presented as an apprentice. On one occasion this deception was thoroughly scuppered as I had committed the gaff of turning up for my day's 'work' wearing a voluminous purple silk shirt; I can still remember my 'gatekeeper's' horror.

Summary and conclusion

The theory of social representations has taken root in social psychology departments. This is as it should be. To reveal the genesis and communication of representations, social psychologists interested in the theory face the challenge of employing qualitative, rather than quantitative, research methodologies. The enduring popularity of quantitative research tools may partly explain why certain social representationalists have shied away from the study of the interplay between rituals and representations. I believe that an understanding of something as complex as the representations expressed and created in current mortuary practices can only be obtained by going into the field and by making use of qualitative research techniques. I would argue that had I used traditional quantitative methodologies, I would not have been able to penetrate this culture of death. Chapter 5, in which I discuss the role of the body and the way our fear of pollution influences our death practices, owes its existence to my participant observational study. While I also illustrate the chapter with quotations gained from interviews, it was my fieldwork observations which alerted me to the existence of our fear of the ambiguous corpse. Much the same happened to Jodelet (1991) in her study of the social representations of mental illness. During her fieldwork she discovered that some of the villagers of the small French community of Ainay-le-Château preferred to use separate sets of cutlery for their mentally ill lodgers, thereby expressing their fear of contamination.

The qualitative study described in some detail in this chapter was designed to help me identify our current social representations of death. I achieved this perspective by means of two quite distinct, yet related, methodologies: participant observation and in-depth interviewing. Such a combination allowed me to verify information, contemporaneously and *in situ*, by referring to alternative sources of data. Yet while I have come to a unique perspective, this perspective is not idiosyncratic. I trust that the scenarios and explanations I have described would be recognizable to any of the actors I observed or spoke to. It is simply that, belonging to only one part of a complex picture, these actors could not have arrived at the same conclusions themselves.

3 Medicine and bureaucracy

Prior (1989) has noted that it is a testament to the complex nature of current mortuary practices that we now need handbooks, such as the Consumers' Association's guide (Rudinger 1986), in order to find our way through the maze of administrative and bureaucratic procedures initiated by a death. In the next two chapters I attempt to give a picture of contemporary death practices in London. By the end of these twin chapters we shall have a clearer idea of the complicated nature of contemporary death.

When someone dies a small drama is set in motion. The key players are the deathwork professionals, the grieving next of kin and the corpse itself. In the first few busy days after a death the corpse passes through medical, bureaucratic, commercial and ritual domains. While there is a great deal of overlap and to-ing and fro-ing between these domains, it is easy to see that the social organization of death is processual. During my time in the field I travelled the whole route, as it were, moving between frontstage and backstage areas. I was able to get a broader picture than that gained by a grieving relative or someone whose job is connected with the disposal of the dead. The descriptive account that follows reveals the points of view of both the deathwork professional and that of their grieving 'client'.

> To talk of the organisation of death is therefore to talk of the body of rules and practices through which human actors relate to death at both a physical and theoretical level. The rules are contained and expressed in and through conversations, behaviour, manuals of procedure, text-books, death certificates and the like, and they are composed and utilised in specific sites or settings. And, put together, one can see that these diverse and varied elements form a discourse on death, a discourse which defines the very nature and meaning of mortality in the modern world.
>
> (Prior 1989: 200)

In an inspiring study of the social organization of death in Belfast, Prior looked at the ways in which discourses of death are used to socially organize this biological event. He shows how 'disease and death are not referents about which there are discourses but objects constructed by discourse' (Prior 1989: 3). This point of view informed the research described in the next two chapters.

Death and the medical model

Since 1945, the biomedical model of disease has been the dominant influence in the practice of medicine and the education of its practitioners. In this model, disease is defined as physical and biochemical deviations from established norms, and the body is treated as a broken machine subject to recovery through replacement or repair of defective body parts.

(Benoliel and Degner 1995: 120)

Field (1996) notes that the process of dying has become an institutional and medicalized event, with nurses and doctors playing an important and powerful role in most people's experiences of dying. This was certainly supported by my own research. Many of my bereaved respondents' accounts of their partners' deaths were dominated by descriptions of their interactions with medical and nursing staff and the hospital or hospice in which their relative was a patient. Even the home deaths were, to varying degrees, medical events.

While sudden death has always been part of the human condition, dying over a longer period of time as the result of chronic illness and the deterioration of ageing is a singularly twentieth-century phenomenon. The experience of dying in hospital has changed with the 'industrialisation of disease management and death control' (Benoliel and Degner 1995: 120). They argue that 'the practice of medicine has come to be structured and organised around the primacy of the cure ethic' (1995: 124).

Bauman (1992b) argues that the modern era's battle against disease represents an effort to move towards a rhetoric of 'uncertainty of outcome' (1992b: 130). When we come to speak to the dying we talk of their terminal illness and how to fight it. Talk about death is transformed into 'the language of survival' (1992b: 130), and dying becomes an extended negotiation in which a person's mortality is contingent on the success of treatment. Bauman called the process the deconstruction of mortality. One side-effect of the denial of mortality (Becker 1973), this fight for life at all costs, is the way in which death has become hidden. Ironically, this obsession with mortal diseases has permeated life itself as we have become preoccupied with health in a dietary and fitness war against the various causes of death.

Bauman's conception of the modern business of dying often helped me to understand my respondents' descriptions of their husbands' deaths. These were 'revealed' deaths in which treatment had 'failed'. Some women felt bitter and betrayed. Their consultant had let them down, their husbands' bodies had proved to be too weak, the treatment had been applied too late or too poorly. Indeed, even in these times of enlightenment regarding palliative care of the dying person I found that the accounts of loss and bereavement were still spoiled by a description of medical staff battling against death.

Back in 1989, Field bemoaned the 'widespread failure of hospital staff to provide patients with information about their condition'. In my study I also came across instances in which communication was poor. Bert, a retired window cleaner, had cancer of the colon. A few weeks before his death he went into his local hospital for surgery. Doris was dismayed to find her convalescing husband to be extremely poorly. She said she had presumed that the surgery would make him better. She looked to the doctors for further medical intervention and was shocked when she found they were expecting him to die. As far as Doris's conception of medical care went, surgery led to recovery. It is hard to believe that anyone could have surgery without being told about their condition but Doris stated that neither of them knew why he was having surgery or, for that matter, what disease was attacking him. Even if the couple were given information, it is clear that it was not given well. Here she is talking about a conversation with her husband's consultant some days after his surgery:

> He said, 'Do you know what is the matter with him?' Of course I hadn't thought to ask and nobody had said anything. And apparently he had two growths in the bowel, that had fused.
>
> (Doris)

Palliative care and the hospice movement

Descriptions of the industrialization of medical care do not completely cover the story, however. In Britain today there are other ways of looking after the dying. In my sample there were some fortunate couples for whom the pretence of cure had been dropped by medical staff and success had been reinterpreted as a good manner of dying.

From its inception in the 1960s the hospice movement has had a great impact on our experience of dying, especially when death is from cancer (Field 1996). Indeed, Hockey (1990) argues that cancer deaths undermined the success of the medical model and gave rise to the felt need for a new way of caring for the dying. Cancer can befall the relatively young, is characterized by a long illness and it is often varied and unpredictable in its nature. The ideology of the hospice movement centres around three core ideas (Field and Johnson 1993): holistic care; multidisciplinary teams who work in a non-hierarchical fashion; and the incorporation of the family of the patient as part of the unit to receive care. Efforts are made to address the fears and anxieties of the dying person and to care for them in a caring and affectionate environment (Lattanzi-Licht and Connor 1995). Hospices often rely heavily on volunteers, mostly women who have experienced a bereavement themselves. As Field and Johnson (1993) note, however, these ideals are constantly being corroded by the development of larger institutions with their associated needs for more bureaucracy, greater formality and the promotion of status differentiation between staff (see James and Field 1992).

As a better understanding of the process of dying was reached, the care of the dying as a specialism developed within the medical sciences (see Clark 1993). The discipline of palliative medicine emerged in the late 1980s and was only recently recognized by the Royal College of Physicians. While palliative medicine focuses on the physiological symptoms associated with advanced diseases and conditions preceding death, palliative care has more holistic goals, aiming at increasing the dying person's comfort and, thereby, at improving the quality of their life. Interventions include pain control and symptom management, as well as the more ethereal issues of spiritual and emotional health, sharing many of the aspirations of the hospice movement.

In 1994 a book by Nuland, a doctor working in the United States, impressively entitled *How We Die*, was published in Britain with a flurry of publicity. This book explicitly sets out to empower the dying patient, giving graphic and detailed accounts of various terminal conditions such as heart disease, old age, AIDS and cancer in the form of moving personal anecdotes from Nuland's professional life. These accounts are full of medical facts, yet remain essentially humanistic. For example, in an echo of Elias's (1985) call for an end to the loneliness of dying, Nuland states in his concluding chapter that 'death belongs to the dying and those who love them' (Nuland 1994: 265). His book neatly reflects the fine balance we struggle to achieve between the aspiration of personal empowerment and the seduction of medical interventions.

There was evidence to suggest that the partners of the middle-class respondents in my study attempted to appropriate their own deaths. Eleanor's husband's response to hearing a bad prognosis on his condition – cancer of the prostate – was to call up a friend of his who was a consultant oncologist. The three of them spent the evening together talking about the likely progression of the disease and its symptoms. Similarly, Ann felt her husband broke out of a severe bout of depression exacerbated by his first course of chemotherapy after he had asked a medical friend to come over for a chat about his dying trajectory. These men were active in the decision-making process regarding when to start opiate-based drugs to relieve their pain. Both men were busy tidying-up loose ends in their work and were keen not to lose the ability to think clearly. When they were too poorly to make their own decisions, their wives took over the role, weighing carefully the benefits and costs of pain relief. The women's accounts gave me a strong impression of families being in control over the death of one of their members. My respondents' active role in the care of their dying husbands was clearly identified as a source of pride and comfort. While still relying heavily on the support and advice of medical practitioners, they felt they had been in charge and in control. Their close involvement in the dying process seemed to ease them into the first hours of their bereavements. Ann's husband died at dawn and throughout the rest of the day she would pop in and out of his bedroom to gaze at him lying in his bed as she ushered in various friends and family who had come to her house to pay their last respects. She surprised herself with a sense of calm that seemed to bear little resemblance to the numb incomprehension normally associated with an 'early grief reaction'.

Dying

Identifying a person as 'dying' is difficult because it is a cultural construct: a label which marks the shift in expectation from being ill and recovering, to being ill and not recovering. This label is rarely applied lightly, not least because there is no guarantee that the medical personnel will agree on a likely outcome (Benoliel and Degner 1995). Once some kind of consensus has been reached, the clinicians will ideally tell the terminally ill person that they are dying; but even nowadays, people are not always told (Schou 1993; Katz 1993).

In the 1960s Glaser and Strauss went 'into the field' on hospital wards in which patients were dying. Clearly inspired by Durkheim's (1952) collective representations and also explicitly drawing on Van Gennup's (1960) observations regarding 'rites de passage', Glaser and

Strauss (1965) developed a schema in which they could describe the dying patient's status passages from patient to corpse. Focusing on the disclosure of terminal prognosi made by medical staff to their patients they coined the now-familiar phrases 'awareness states' and 'dying trajectories'. Glaser and Strauss suggested that four categories of awareness state exist: closed awareness, suspected awareness, mutual pretence and open awareness. Common sense would suggest that a state of open awareness, in which patients and staff acknowledge the imminent death, would be preferable to remaining in a state of mutual pretence. There may be compelling reasons for non-disclosure, however. Further, there are times when denial is healthy. More than thirty years later the messy mix of awareness states continues to exist. I encountered several instances of closed awareness, in which family, friends and staff became engaged in a conspiracy of silence in order to protect the patient from the news that they would soon be dead.

Three years later Glaser and Strauss released another publication in which they turned their attention to the ways in which we construct various trajectories of dying. For example, as the term implies, a lingering trajectory is characterized by a gradual decline towards death. In contrast, the quick or unexpected trajectory leaves little or no time for preparation. Glaser and Strauss (1968) observed the subtle interplay between staff, patients and next of kin. Everyone constructs different expectations of how the dying trajectory will be expressed and how long it will last. Dying 'too soon', for example, can cause great upset. Christine was angry with her husband's consultant who, she claimed, had changed his prognosis in the space of two days from a year or two's life to that of a matter of weeks. Such was her fury against this particular man that in her descriptions of her husband's demise it is his consultant rather than his cancer that steals years from him.

> I remember the first time they said Alan had two years. But when the doctor saw him the second time, he took me to another room and said he only had about a month. Suddenly only a month. That's a bloody difference between years and then months.
>
> (Christine)

In an ideal scenario, the unique dying trajectory of the patient is carefully observed and contained by a palliative care team who maintain a steady flow of information to the dying person and their next of kin. Following a 'treatment trajectory', the patient may undergo surgery while symptoms of their condition are controlled, as much as possible, by drugs or treatments such as radiation or physiotherapy.

Particularly towards the end of a life, people suffering from a variety of progressive diseases or conditions should be able to expect the palliation of their symptoms (Field 1996).

In the last twenty years the process of dying has attracted a great deal of research. Most famous among the early studies inspired by developments within the hospice movement was Kubler-Ross's (1970, 1975) work on the stages of dying. She suggested that her respondents travelled a path through emotional states that, ideally, led to their acceptance of death. During their journey towards death they experienced progressive stages of denial, anger, bargaining and depression. Despite its enduring popularity, this model of dying as some kind of linear process has had its critics. For example, Littlewood (1992) argues that this stage–phase view of the business of dying has the potential to pathologize those who do not adhere to the constructed 'norm'.

Mulkay (1993) draws attention to the uncomfortable topic of social death. Hidden behind the apparent improvements to the pattern of mortality, in which the very elderly make a sedate and gradual decline into death, we can identify a trend in which the social existence of the dying person is 'often reduced, and sometimes more or less eliminated, in the hospital setting owing to other parties' physical, emotional and communicative withdrawal' (1993: 32). Support for this thesis is provided by Field who found that terminally ill patients became passive receivers of expert care and that there was a general 'neglect of the patient as a person' (1989: 147).

> I often see patients who are dying. They are put into a side ward and they will be watching the doctors doing their round and they will say to me 'The doctor hasn't been in to see me for several days. Why is that?'
>
> (Sharon, Sister)

Of course, understanding people's fears of abandonment has to be balanced against the need to give them the space to die (Samerel 1995). Samerel warns that a dying person may appear detached, during which time they may well review their life and prepare for the journey into death; the dying person is often psychologically disengaging with the world of the living. Death is also a physical event and the symptoms of dying may simply preoccupy the dying person. People may display all or a mixture of the following bodily symptoms: loss of muscle tone, dysphasia, dysphagia, decreased gastrointestinal activity, decreased sphincter control, sluggish circulation, changes in vital signs (such as blood pressure) and sensory impairment (Samerel 1995). With experience medical staff learn to recognize the signficance of these symptoms and can predict that death is near.

Social death and social value are closely linked. In a society that worships youth, the socially valuable members of society are the young and reproductively active. Blauner (1966) suggested that we can observe very different responses to the deaths of those apparently high status individuals when compared to the under-valued. The chronically sick, disabled or elderly receive lower quality care while they are dying, cause less urgent life-saving efforts at the moment of death and create less of a stir when dead.

> [We feel worse] if they are young, like someone [who dies] giving birth by a Caesarean, or someone who has died a couple of days after a massive car crash. Because in fact, life is more sacred, I suppose, when you are younger. Obviously. Much cheaper when you are old.
>
> (Charlotte, Doctor)

It is easy to see why relations between patients, kin and staff are not always harmonious. In a study of the experience of parents whose children had cancer Ball *et al.* (1996) found that every meeting between medical practitioner and parent was coloured with the possibilities of either hearing good or bad news. They noted a situation of 'heightened cue awareness' in which worried parents analysed and over-interpreted everything that was said and done by the staff. These exchanges can be vividly remembered. During my research I was constantly surprised to find that my respondents recalled lengthy conversations with medical personnel.

Expected death in the hospital ward

If a death is expected and if the patient is staying in a hospital ward or at a hospice, every effort is made to ensure that the immediate family are present at the moment of death. Emergency telephone numbers of next of kin are collected by the sister on the ward. Some hospitals and hospices have facilities for relatives to live in guest rooms or, alternatively, close relatives may camp by the patient's bed during the final few days or hours. If a patient cannot be moved to a private room the curtains round the bed act as a fragile barrier to the outside world, blocking out the curious, sympathetic or fearful gaze of fellow patients.

During such bedside vigils, it can be quite hard for medical staff to create the kind of backstage environment in which their work is made more comfortable and easy (Goffmann 1961). Staff can suggest to weary relatives that they take a tea break or a walk. Or relatives may simply be asked to leave the room while certain procedures take place. There are signs that such attitudes are changing, however. Nurses in many wards now encourage relatives to take an active part in caring for the dying patient. They may be shown how to clean and moisten their dying relative's mouth, for example.

If the relatives are present when the patient dies they are usually guided through the death by one nurse who has been assigned to them. If an empathic relationship has developed these nurses can play an extraordinarily important role. Without any obvious formalized training or the help of debriefing or counselling, these professionals bear tremendous emotional strain. Nursing the terminally ill is a stressful job and working conditions can be difficult. Staff are 'overworked, exploited and unsupported' (Field 1989: 147). Katz (1996) found that nurses who looked after terminally ill patients on a cancer ward found their source of stress was not the death of the patient so much as their ability to maintain good nursing standards. This is dependent on external factors such as ward management and relationships with doctors and other medical staff.

Hospital clergy are also there to provide pastoral care. They play an extraordinary role looking after the spiritual health of hundreds of patients, some of whom are dying. Their aspirations for the spiritual health of patients often exists uneasily within the medical model.

> There are tricks of the trade, if one can put it like that. For example, if we were asked to visit a particular patient who was known to be dying we wouldn't march straight up to the bed because there is all this sort of folklore about the clergyman being, you know, the Angel of Death on the ward.
>
> (The Reverend Ralph Peters)

Imminent death is relatively easy to identify as it is physiologically signposted by dilated and fixed pupils; an inability to move; loss of reflexes; weaker, more rapid pulse; Cheyne-Stokes respirations; noisy breathing; and lowered blood pressure (Samerel 1995). Death follows a predictable flow from heart stoppage, the end of respiration and the death of the brain (Veatch 1995). But in a society in which technological advances have opened up a debate into the very definition of death itself, deciding that someone has died is not necessarily a simple task. The ancient criteria of signs of breath and heartbeat have turned to more recent questions of brain function (Zucker 1995). As Veatch notes, 'society used to believe that persons with beating heart were alive even though their brain function was lost irreversibly. Now society is not so sure' (1995: 405). In fact, someone who is breathing and whose heart is still beating thanks to the life-support system they are dependent upon, can be defined as dead if they are also found to be in a permanently vegetative state.

Discussions still rage as to whether this definition of brain death should include whole brain or just the centres of higher function. These debates extend from the territory of biology to social philosophy and cause us to consider the moral rights of individuals (Zucker 1995). Ideally, the definition of death would be left somewhat flexible, viewed as a process rather than a state. At times it is more useful to simply consider the quality of life left to the critically ill patient, rather than to struggle in the morass of death definitions (Veatch 1995). But these issues may not have become so important had it not been for the tremendous value, and shortage, of organs and tissues for transplantation (Veatch 1995). Further, in our litigatious society precise definitions are needed in order to protect the rights of both the dying and those who care for them. In response to these complex questions, many dying patients choose to execute living wills in which they state their preferences regarding life-prolonging procedures when their time for dying comes (Scheible Wolf 1995).

Medical crisis: the unexpected or sudden death

Serious accidents or sudden critical illness lead to a completely different experience for the dying, and for those close to them, than a slow and expected decline. Death becomes an emergency situation in which there is a rush to get the dying or dead person to the local hospital's accident and emergency centre. Efforts may be focused on life-saving, even when death seems inevitable. Pappas (1996) notes that the rapid pace of technological advance in medicine is constantly posing new and difficult legal and moral questions regarding medical aid in dying. At what point do heroic life-saving efforts stop? Medical treatments that postpone inevitable death can cause a conflict of interest between the incapacitated patient's right to die with dignity and medical professionalism's very human desire to fight death (Scheible Wolf 1995).

In such situations, relatives may or may not be present. If they are present they may also be injured or suffering from shock. The very nature of life-saving activity precludes the possibility of lengthy interactions between medical personnel and waiting relatives, let alone the critically ill patient who, even if they were conscious at the time of arrival, are likely to be rapidly sedated (Benoliel and Degner 1995). The supply of clear information, and with it the opportunity to prepare for death and to say goodbye can, quite understandably, go out of the window.

> When you're involved in acute emergency situations then I think it is impractical for the relatives to be there. Because I think they couldn't cope with it. And I think the staff would find it very difficult to function, too.
>
> (John, intensive care unit nurse)

Reg, who had a history of heart disease, was admitted to hospital after feeling 'poorly'. In the quotation that follows, Paula is describing what happened just after he had been admitted.

> I was standing at the side of him, talking to him like this. And all of a sudden he just made this odd gurgling noise and went. And I sort of stood for a moment. I sort of stared at him, I don't know what I thought I was doing. I very calmly turned round and said to the doctor 'I think my husband has died.' When you look back you wonder why you do these things. And of course, he sort of spun round and the next thing I knew [I was] thrown out and there were nurses and doctors rushing in, like a scene from television. They came from every direction, I have never seen anyone move so fast.
>
> (Paula)

This resuscitation attempt was 'successful' and a bewildered Paula was reintroduced to Reg. After a couple of hours she was sent home by Reg himself who had poignantly muttered to her that 'a fellow couldn't get any rest'. Shortly after she had left the hospital Reg suffered another heart attack. This time he could not be brought back to life.

Until recently, it has been accepted policy to remove relatives during a resuscitation attempt. The assumption has been that violent and hasty activity would be distressing to relatives. There have also been fears that emotional bystanders could get in the way of the lifesavers. So generally, if the resuscitation team are called, relatives are hauled out of the way. As is the case now in many aspects of our death and dying customs, this over-protective attitude is being questioned. It is possible that much of our institutionalized protection may be serving the deathwork professional better than the dying or grieving public.

Intensive care units provide another stage for dying the modern death. The focus in such units is on preventing death in the critically ill. Organ failure and rapid death is a constant threat and medical staff have to remain alert for the signs of decline, ready to move fast. Under such emergency conditions there can be little allowance for patient privacy or easy access for relatives (Benoliel and Degner 1995). Despite the efforts of staff to both save life and preserve the dignity of the ill patient, dying in intensive care is undoubtedly depersonalizing.

> Those who die there generally end their lives attached to all manner of life-prolonging apparatus, and often death occurs after intensive heroic activity by the staff. Dying in the intensive care unit is one of the new rituals of transition in a technologically sophisticated society, and it makes the central participant something of an object.
>
> (Benoliel and Degner 1995: 130)

Once it is clear that a patient is not going to live then the possibility of obtaining organs for donation arises. Negotiating with relatives on this matter is highly stressful; the issue of 'organ harvesting' is complex (see Richardson 1996). Robbins (1996) found that relatives were sometimes very disturbed by requests for organs. This reaction can partly be explained by the fact that such requests often represent the first moment when relatives truly realize that death has occurred. The difficulties are further exacerbated because the next of kin are not always present when the life-support machine is finally turned off after the removal of the donated organs. The removal of corneas, for example, can leave the face quite disfigured. However strong the argument that the patient is already dead, relatives still appear to view the moment of switching off the machine at the moment of death. This is not surprising. The cutting of electricity means that the chest no longer lifts and sinks and the heartbeat stops.

The dead patient

Once someone has been pronounced dead, behaviour towards the body undergoes a dramatic change. As Veatch (1995) notes, we have a totally different set of social behaviours towards the newly dead to

that of the dying. In short, the social system of death behaviour is set
in motion. If the relatives are not present at the moment of death,
nursing staff will make efforts to tidy-up the body before their arrival.
The hair is brushed, the face may be washed and the body straightened
into a reposeful position. The bed is remade and drips and syringes
may be removed. Being with the body, immediately after death, while
it is still warm, is clearly important to grieving relatives. This is a
point when the inert body still looks and smells familiar. However, in
busy NHS hospitals, staff may find themselves pressed to find the time
to prepare the body for relatives. Ruth waited three and a half hours
before she was able to see her husband in the frantic casualty department where his body had been taken after his death in the street.

> I was put into a small room, to wait. We waited there, without
> anybody saying anything to us, or coming to us, from about
> twelve to half-past three. And that I found objectionable . . .
> Of course they were busy in casualty. But I wouldn't have minded
> to have seen my husband with his torn clothes. They obviously
> had to cut clothes off him, to try to put the machines on him to
> try and get his heart going again . . . I wouldn't have minded
> that. I mean, what is wrong with, with a cut anorak. Why they,
> apparently stripped him and just put him under a sheet for me to
> see. I found that a bit curious . . . if you have lived for forty years
> with someone, you don't mind seeing a torn anorak, you know?
> (Ruth)

People are usually left with the body for a while. This period of time
seems subject to the personal taste of the sister in charge. The same
element of chance creeps in with the decision of how many grieving
relatives are allowed around the death bed. In London hospitals
'normal behaviour' has been modelled on a Christian nuclear family.
'Next of kin' means spouse, parents and children. In those cultures
that encourage close ties with an extended family, next of kin also
includes cousins, aunts, uncles and grand-parents. This can mean that
a large party turns up to pay their last respects. In one hospital where I
carried out fieldwork I did detect efforts to understand these cultural
differences even though staff tended to grumble about the more
expressive grief of sizeable gatherings of Bengali or Greek mourners
(see Gardner 1998).

Leaving a hospital ward as grieving next of kin, possibly after weeks
of great emotional intensity, can be difficult. Strong, dependent
relationships may have been forged with staff. Having been the centre

of attention the bereaved may become aware of their redundancy on the ward. Certainly the women I spoke to expressed an overwhelming urge to remain with the body. So, in addition to the trauma of the death, relatives have to cope with this sudden physical separation from the corpse.

> And then we left the ward. And I had the feeling that they wanted to get rid of us, they wanted to sort of bundle us out of the hospital. Which rather surprised me. I sort of thought, well, perhaps, shall we stay until the morning? Obviously they didn't want that.
>
> (Margaret)

They also experience a great change in status as they are now tainted with death. Staff freely admit that the relatives' grief can be personally upsetting and nurses I spoke to talked of their feeling of impotency when faced with this rude reminder of sorrow and loss. In open wards, nurses may also be concerned for the feelings of their surviving patients. I am sure it can be harrowing to be lying next to a death-bed scene if one is poorly. If the death had been preceded by a resuscitation attempt or a long battle to save the life of the patient, the medical staff may feel the sight of a crying relative as a recrimination. As they battle with feelings of personal failure, perhaps it is no surprise that doctors may sometimes act like the proverbial cat on a hot tin roof.

> Then you say goodbye to the relatives, who invariably ask you 'So, what do we do now?' and I go 'I don't know, it's not really my job to deal with that, it's the relative liaison officer's.'
>
> (Charlotte, Doctor)

> I think [the doctors are] scared of patients dying . . . because a lot of people expect doctors to cure. And a lot of doctors see it as a failure. They have failed. Which is absolutely ridiculous . . . and I think they find it hard to go to the relatives.
>
> (Sharon, Sister)

Once the relatives have left, the nursing staff prepare the body for its removal to the mortuary. In line with the military style of traditional nursing, nurses used to be expected to 'lay-out' the body, which involved plugging orifices and binding limbs. Nowadays nursing staff merely wash the body and put it in a body bag.

Continuing the theme of privacy, one sister on a surgical ward explained how she puts curtains around all the other beds in the ward to spare the surviving patients the distressing site of the body being removed in a covered mortuary trolley. The curtains again act as a barometer of what is acceptable in a public space.

It is possible to view bodies in hospital chapels or in the mortuary, although many people choose to say their goodbyes at the bedside. If relatives were not there at the time of death then they can get access to their late kin by visiting the hospital at a prearranged time. For example, one of the widows I interviewed visited the mortuary because she had been abroad at the time of her husband's death. Generally the hospital mortuary is a backstage area, a place where bodies are kept until they are released to the funeral director. Some corpses may undergo a post-mortem for investigative or research purposes. In such instances the relatives are either asked or informed prior to the post-mortem.

Unlike the viewing at the funeral parlour, in which great care is made to make the body 'presentable', a body viewed in the mortuary or at a viewing chapel may not be prepared for the visitors. Although the hair may be brushed, face washed and the corpse may be dressed, the body is not embalmed and it is unlikely that make-up will be applied. For example, when Beth went to visit her husband at the hospital she found the experience 'not terribly pleasant'. The following is taken from my fieldnotes:

> The viewing chapel is situated in the bowels of the hospital building. This chapel [looks as if it] has not been redecorated since the 1960s. It is an airless, practically windowless room (just grating glass under a pavement) and all dark red velvet and dark wood, like a chapel. Oppressive, hot and airless, with an unpleasant smell of air freshener . . . It seemed such a poor and alien place to see someone you loved.
>
> (Fieldnotes, hospital viewing chapel)

Relatives often name the hospital as the beneficiary of money at the funeral, in lieu of flowers. They may also choose to have a memorial service at the hospital chapel, although this can be problematic in an institution that is ambivalent about its role in dealing with death. I was told of one instance in which a service for a child who had died was only agreed to by the hospital authorities on condition that the windows were blacked out. It was felt that a memorial service would be bad for morale.

Expected deaths at home

Increasingly, people choose to die at home. There are many advantages to a home death as it often allows family members to play a central role in the care of the dying person. There are also some disadvantages, however. Field states that 'care of the sick and dying in the community is not keeping pace with the increased demand for services' (1989: 148). Bowling and Cartwright (1982) found home care of the dying was often poor. Without good support it can be very demanding for relatives. Despite the fact that she was very well supported by friends and a terminal support team, Ann did not take a break from caring for her husband for weeks on end. Another women, who was quite elderly, found that she could not cope with the physical demands of looking after her very sick husband. She was relieved when he was finally moved to a local hospice.

Providing care-givers are given adequate support, an expected death at home can be positive. Of course the medical team's control of the situation is made more tenuous because they are not in their own space. Just as it can be hard for medical personnel to create a backstage environment in front of a family who have set up a bedside vigil in the ward, palliative nurses and other visiting health professionals may find there are times when they also want to work backstage. Space can be created by asking relatives to leave or by simply slipping into speech that is full of medical jargon. Alternatively, the palliative care team may step back and leave the care of the dying person to the family. Ball *et al.* (1996) found that parents of children with cancer often took over the management of care as a natural extension of their parenting role. As they note, this 'naturalisation of death' in a family and home setting runs counter to current stereotypes of dying as a technical or institutionalized event.

> The nurse explained everything, she had said what would happen to him, so I knew from the Friday, when she told me, what would happen. But, even so, even though she'd said what would happen – with the rattle and all that – it still shocks you. So, when it started I knew exactly, I knew exactly what was happening but it still shocks you when it happens.
>
> (Christine)

Modern terminal support teams, inspired by the hospice movement, can help orchestrate moving death-bed scenes. Ball *et al.* note that paediatric oncology nurses can act as stage-managers (1996). I came across two examples of such deaths. While there still may be a medical sub-text to these home deaths, with the administration of powerful pain-killing drugs, they are different because the relatives can remain with the body after the death. It is the medical staff who leave, not the relatives.

After an expected death at home the family's GP will visit the body to ascertain the cause of death before contacting a second GP, who also has to see the corpse. The funeral director then comes to the house to remove the body.

Sudden death and 'death messages'

Not all deaths occur in a medical setting. People can die suddenly for a variety of reasons and in all sorts of unexpected places. If a death is not preceded by a long illness then it is regarded as a 'sudden death' by the police. Most 'sudden deaths', however, are not dramatic, befalling elderly people who die in their homes (Mitchell 1996). If the doctor called to the scene is unable to ascertain a straightforward cause of death then the body becomes the possession of the coroner who can order a post-mortem. The corpse may be held as 'evidence' as part of a police investigation. The police also become involved when violent and/or dramatic incidents occur such as road-traffic and building-site accidents, homicide, suicide, drug overdose and cot death. These unplanned and unexpected events pose real challenges to the system.

As Mitchell (1996) notes, police-training manuals emphasize the need for entering into any sudden death situation with an open mind. The scene of death may also be a scene of crime. It may be necessary for the police to seal-off an area around the body for forensic investigation. Relatives may be shocked to find that they cannot get access to the body immediately after the death if it has to be photographed and examined. If relatives are present, the police may need to interview them not only as witnesses but also as potential suspects. One police officer told me of the difficulties of gently interrogating an outwardly calm mother whose baby had died in suspicious circumstances. A father of a child the same age as the dead baby, he found himself caught with ambivalent feelings of angry suspicion and understandable sympathy aroused by the tragic situation.

If relatives are not present then the police become involved in delivering 'death messages'. This is not a popular chore. My police respondents unequivocally described this as a dire and distressing task and could vividly describe vignettes of 'breaking bad news' many years after the event; these were quite clearly upsetting memories.

> I knew when the doorbell rang. I hadn't opened the door yet. The doorbell rang, and I thought, 'So. And now you are going to be told that he is dead.' And I opened the door, there was the policeman and I said 'My husband is dead.' And he said 'Yes.' There was no reason, but I knew. I think we all have instincts in us, if we let them, you know, talk to us.
>
> (Ruth)

> Everyone automatically assumes that police officers get this fantastic training on how to break this terrible news, you know, that their kids have been run over by trucks . . . I certainly have never had any. You know, as a young probationary constable, I can remember years ago, being sent out to go and tell Mrs Smith her son has died, or that her husband won't be coming home. And you think 'Great, how do I go about it.'
>
> (Inspector Brown)

The police involved in the breaking of bad news may then accompany the relatives to the mortuary to view the body. If the body needs to be viewed for identification purposes there may be a clash of purpose between the shocked relative and the police conducting the viewing. While the relative may wish to say goodbye, the police may wish for the viewing to be carried out as rapidly as possible. Things are made even more complicated if the body is mutilated. Professionals, such as police, doctors or coroners, often feel that only certain categories of family members, usually male, are up to the task of seeing it.

> There are circumstances where it would be, I think, asking too much of a person who is not professionally concerned with the mutilated dead to look at somebody who has been damaged in a road traffic, rail accident, burnt, drowned and remained in the water until the body has been totally disfigured. At that point, we say no, we will have to have a secondary form of identification . . . There is always a margin, where, well, he is a policeman, alright, he can see his wife, sister, daughter, who is a bit, a bit damaged, but it is all in a day's work for him, he doesn't have to but, you know, macho man and all that, people in the fire service and stuff like that I think would insist on doing it. We prefer, obviously we prefer, but we are still an exclusively male outlet here and we

reckon identifying bodies is a male job. So we would rather call a brother-in-law, than a wife. You see?

(Coroner)

Disfigured bodies were still deeply shocking to the professionals. It was interesting to see how they claimed to resort to humour in the face of decapitations and such like. Apparently there are some 'old favourites' which are talked about during training. I was told of a couple of these tales that, apparently, help the police to cope with the stressful situations in which they find themselves. I remain sceptical whether they were ever told as jokes, largely because they do not seem funny. Mitchell (1996) notes that there has been an assumption that the use of black humour represents one of the coping strategies resorted to by the police in the 'tough culture' that demands a calm response to shocking incidents, but she found little evidence that gallows humour was resorted to as a helpful coping strategy.

Unexpected deaths rarely facilitate the kind of calm that can be generated in an expected death. As some of my respondent's accounts poignantly illustrate, the whole experience of bereavement may be skewed by the memory of panic, shock and fear. Mitchell (1996) notes there has been an assumption that the trauma of sudden deaths mostly affects the next of kin. But research (Duckworth 1986) suggests that police officers and other professionals also suffer great distress when unexpectedly faced with a dead body.

Relatives find that they spend most of the period immediately after a death coming into contact with a variety of medical personnel. Within hours of the death, there is a shift from those people who try to stop or control death to those people who are responsible for inventorying the dead and their property. The bereaved relatives are now entering a phase of bureaucracy.

The coroner

The coroner's court looks as if it were built at the end of the last century. An austere, red brick building with a small court and offices. This small court is built away from the road and it was quite hard to find . . . One enters the building through a side door, and having passed through a rather dank corridor (there is a strong smell of disinfectant) I found myself in front of the reception. This office seems to have become stuck in a time warp – circa 1950. Ancient typewriters sit on outdated office desks. To my surprise the clerks used huge leather-bound books, in which they

make their entries. The clerks were joking around. One of the
clerks sauntered up to the 'reception' and asked me what I
wanted.
I was shown through to the coroner's office. Which, I suppose,
few relatives actually get to see. This old room was a total mess,
piles of yellowing papers and files stacked on the floor. A large old
desk flooded with correspondence, files and books and littered
with old coffee cups. Sitting in front of his desk, I could hardly see
him over the debris.

(Fieldnotes, coroner's office)

A coroner becomes involved if the cause of death is sudden, unclear or
if the circumstances surrounding the death give rise to suspicion of
foul play. If the coroner believes that someone was killed, they will
open the inquest, identify the deceased and then hand the case over to
the criminal prosecution service (Hallam *et al.* forthcoming).

Coroners are usually drawn from the medical profession and have
full control over the corpse. It is a prestigious job and of all the
professionals involved in the social organization of death, the coroner
appears to enjoy the highest status. Coroners may become involved in
the viewing of the body by relatives for identification purposes. As we
can see from the quotation in the previous section, the coroner I
interviewed had very strong opinions about which gender was more
able to cope with the identification of bodies. This was most definitely
man's work. Mitchell (1994) identified similar gender assumptions in
her study of people's perceived ability to cope with traumatic incidents.

The rate of referrals to the coroner is steadily increasing. Home
Office figures reveal that in 1920 11 per cent of deaths were referred to
the coroner; by 1970 the figure had risen to 23 per cent. In 1997, 35
per cent of deaths were reported to the coroner. It is the coroner's job
to order a post-mortem to ascertain the cause of death. It is a coroner
who orders a hospital pathologist to carry out a post-mortem,
although consultants may approach relatives independently to request
permission to carry out a post-mortem for medical research purposes.
Even though the relatives may not have very much contact with the
coroner, his involvement has direct repercussions for them as it may
cause a delay of the funeral. If the coroner is investigating the cause
of death then we can expect delays in the issuing of the death
certificate and the release of the body for burial or cremation. Every
effort is made to keep these delays to a minimum. However, in cases of
murder or suspected murder the body may be held in a mortuary for

many months so that an accused person can apply for an independent post-mortem.

On the basis of the post-mortem and police reports, coroners may choose to order an inquest into the cause of death. In an inner-city coroner's office about 20 per cent of referrals end up in an inquest. Given the complex social problems facing the capital, this rate is understandably higher than many rural areas which remain constant at about 10 per cent. Inquests can take place with or without a jury.

In an inquest the coroner will undertake a delicate balancing act between the social and medical causes of death (Prior 1989). The police are primarily interested in unearthing the social causes of death. In a car accident their focus is not so much on the medical cause of death but on the behaviour of the driver concerned as well as other contextual factors such as the road conditions, the presence of other drivers or unforeseen obstacles in the road. The coroner attempts to marry the evidence from the pathologist's post-mortem report – medical – with that of the evidence supplied by the police and other witnesses – social. As the sole purpose of an inquest is to investigate the cause of death, not to attribute blame, the products of such a marriage are often weird sociolegal descriptions of death, such as 'accident or misadventure' (which described 47 per cent of deaths in one particular London court in 1997) or 'death by natural causes' (describing 13 per cent of inquest verdicts).

As few of us know the exact definition of such terms, we may remain in the dark as to the true cause of death. The vagueness of the 'cause of death' and the non-accusatory stance adopted by coroners can cause feelings of bitterness among relatives who are eager to find out who was responsible for their loved one's demise. Hallam *et al.* (forthcoming) note the divergence in perspectives that arises in the course of an inquest, as expert and lay witnesses describe how and why the death occurred. While the pathologist's report, perceived in court as 'inherently objective, learned and scientific', is viewed as the truth that will lead to a closure of the case, lay accounts focus on the need to explain the death in the context of their continuing, bereaved, lives.

The patients' affairs officer

The Hospital Administration Department is sited in an overcrowded warren of small offices on the third floor. The bereaved have to pass along a corridor from which the various offices lead. You enter and find yourself in a tiny 'waiting room' with a row of orange soft chairs and a coffee table. Lined up against the wall are hospital posters and row upon row of leaflets on *What to do when someone dies*. Her office, which she shares with another secretary, leads off from the waiting space. The office is chaotic. Lined up against one wall were a row of black poly bags with deceaseds' belongings – this is dreary . . . Medics, who have been asked to fill in the Death Certificate and the Certificate for Cremation, wander in and out.

(Fieldnotes, patients' affairs office)

If a death took place in a hospital then relatives may meet the patients' affairs officer. In many ways these officers bridge the gap between the medical world of the hospital and the bureaucratic world of the registrar's office. It is this person's job to return the deceased's belongings to the family. They also hand over the double-signed certificate of cause of death. This usually takes place the day after the death.

Each morning Trish, a patients' affairs officer in a busy London hospital, was given the medical files and the belongings of those patients who had died the day before. Having skimmed the file to find the cause of death written down by the first doctor who certified the death and having logged in the patient's clothes and valuables, she would then begin to chase up those young doctors who had agreed, for a nominal fee, to sign the second half of the certificate of cause of death. Trish had a list of 'ash cash' doctors pinned above her desk. Chasing up overworked doctors, getting them to examine the body and sign the form was, she claimed, her biggest headache. Next came her battle with doctors to use 'acceptable' causes of death. Like dishonoured cheques, death certificates are 'bounced' by the registrar if doctors use certain social, rather than medical, explanations for cause of death. Saying a person died of 'old age', or as a result of 'smoking' for example, would be unacceptable so Trish vetted all certificates.

The most difficult, but also according to Trish rewarding, aspect of the patients' affairs officer's job is meeting the bereaved relatives. It is not easy to be faced with a blood-stained, yet familiar, article of clothing the day after a tragic death. Even relatives of patients who were predicted to die for some time are liable to become very upset when faced with a pair of pyjamas. Here, Susan is describing her harrowing appointment with the patients' affairs officer after the tragic death of her husband in a car accident.

She said 'First of all, his possessions, his money' . . . So there was money, and his wallet, and his watch and his Swiss army knife.

And the things from which he was never separated. And, er, very
unexpectedly sort of presented [them] to us.

(Susan)

Having signed the forms to release the possessions, Trish handed over
the sealed envelope containing the certificate of cause of death,
addressed to the registrar. The relatives now have to meet their next
bureaucrat.

The registrar

The main entrance is off to the side of the building, and you have
to ask at a main reception desk of the council building before
being directed through some swing doors. As you enter you are
faced by the open-plan waiting room and, on your left, a glassed-
in reception desk. Looking over the receptionist's shoulder you
can see an open-plan office, where various secretaries are working
and you can hear their chat and laughter as you sit waiting. The
waiting area is basically a hallway and is marked off by the placing
of orange chairs in a square, facing each other. This means that
each person is forced to sit opposite someone else.

(Fieldnotes, register office)

Having obtained a double-signed certificate of cause of death from the
hospital or if the death took place at home, from the family GP, the
bereaved relatives are instructed to take this form to their local register
office, where the registrar notes the details of the death before releasing the official death certificate. The two different types of death
certificate cause a certain amount of confusion for the bereaved.
Although they are not meant to look at the certificate of cause of
death supplied by medical personnel, I was told that most envelopes
arrive at the register office opened. The bereaved are expected to
register the death within a week, although generally people register
the death the very next day. Just as the dead are not seen as dead until
a doctor has certified them as dead, a death is not bureaucratically
recognized as a death until the registrar has released the death certificate. Without this essential piece of paper it is not possible to start
the probate process.

Among the queue of people waiting to register births, marriages
and deaths we can usually spot those who are registering a death. In
addition to their sad or serious demeanour, they often carry the

hospital's polythene bags full of the deceased's belongings. One registrar waxed eloquent on this issue:

> Somebody is sitting in the waiting room, they are waiting, they have their little bag there and obviously we know what the bag is. And the bag falls open and a bedroom slipper falls out or something like that, you know? It must be terrible for them. Surely there must be a more dignified way of passing on these possessions?
>
> (Registrar)

This registrar strongly believed that those waiting to register a death should be left to wait in private. This theme of segregation regularly arises in the social organization of death.

After waiting for a while one is called up for the interview with the registrar. Registrar's offices tend to be impersonal and drab. The questions put to one about the deceased are generally quite straightforward: date of birth, last address, occupation, occupation of husband and the like. Registrars take their job seriously.

> The actual registry experience was all right. The registrar was kind, although a little bit patronizing . . . She was very civil. I was quite interested − in an objective sort of way − to see she patronized me, in the way professionals do.
>
> (Susan)

Accuracy is important. This bureaucratic zeal can appear pedantic or trivial to those who, because of the impact of their recent loss, can scarcely concentrate on the simplest of tasks. Registrars' stories about their daily task of extracting socioeconomic details from bereaved people were often scattered with descriptions of hysterical, unreasonable or irrational outbursts.

Administration and probate

At death most adults leave behind a tangle of debts and assets. If the deceased had a will then this document will name an executor. It is the executor's responsibility, aided by a solicitor, to wind up the business and financial affairs of the deceased. This includes inventorying assets and making claims to insurance companies before paying debts, taxes, administrative costs and funeral expenses. The property remaining is then finally free to be distributed to the surviving family and friends according to specifications in the will. This process can take some time. It is easy to see how this complicated business can be made even more troublesome in the case of an intestate estate: one in which no will has been made.

The first few days after the death are a busy time. In addition to dealing with aspects of the probate process, the bereaved relatives may find themselves involved in huge numbers of telephone calls to friends, family and work colleagues. A bereaved women I spoke to said that this dominated their experience of their early days of bereavement.

> At first one is rather excited by it all. You know, all these people coming and everybody saying nice things about Gerald and letters pouring in. I answered 250 letters.
>
> (Beth)

If the death was sudden and unexpected, there may be even more conversations and hastily written notes. Meanwhile, the immediate family are likely to start to receive visitors, as those close to the deceased pay their last respects. All of this is in addition to visits to the hospital-liaison officer, the registrar and the funeral director. The first few days after a death may leave little time for quiet reflection.

Summary and conclusion

With lengthening dying trajectories and innovations in medical science the process of dying is constantly changing. Increasingly, people have become aware of the need to balance our understandable desire to fight death with an acceptance of it as a natural part of life. Thus, we come across descriptions of death in which the dying person and those who love and care for them focus on the palliation of symptoms and face death as squarely as is humanly possible. An exploration of contemporary deaths reveals that this balance is not always achieved; we still find accounts in which an undignified battle against death was fought and lost.

From the moment of death we can identify a shift in behaviour towards the grieving next of kin and the now inert body. While the relatives may suddenly find themselves to be unwanted on the hospital ward, the body becomes an object of investigation. In the days immediately following a death, the body and those who were close to it in life travel along very different routes. The corpse remains in the possession of a string of deathwork professionals. It is kept backstage where it is examined, certified and dressed. Meanwhile, during this harrowing first week, the bereaved relatives trundle from appointment to appointment: picking up the deceased's possessions and registering the death; visiting or contacting the solicitor, bank, insurance companies and social services. In times when many people are often geographically dispersed, relatives also become involved in a huge number of telephone calls to family, friends and work colleagues. Thus, the survivors find themselves embroiled in the very complex business of unravelling the dead person's citizenship.

4   Commerce and ritual

The bereaved client as consumer

However we look at it, the members of the funeral industry, the
florists, funeral directors, cemeteries, crematoria, and those small
manufacturing businesses which supply funerary artefacts such as
coffins, urns, gravestones and memorial plaques, are concerned with
making money. They may do their jobs very well and many of these
workers are compassionate, sensitive and caring. But, ultimately, they
are concerned with profit. Such motives stand in stark contrast to the
medical and administrative staff introduced earlier who are not usually
involved in persuading people to make purchases. When arranging to
dispose of the corpse bereaved people find themselves shopping.

The funeral 'director'

> The Normans' Funeral Parlour can be found in a row of busy,
> prosperous shops in a London street. The frontage stands out in
> so far as it is so drab and old-fashioned. Merely a plate-glass
> window behind which are displayed a bunch of elderly dried
> flowers and a few black and white photographs of old fashioned,
> horse-drawn, funeral cortèges. When you enter, a bell rings by
> the door and a receptionist – male – emerges from the office in
> the back. You are led into a waiting-room. This is a tiny, airless,
> windowless room with an old fashioned Constable print gracing
> one wall. This, along with the floral wall paper and swirly-
> patterned carpets, gives one the distinct feeling that one has
> entered an old people's home. Everything feels rather out of date
> and a bit run down. You are offered a cup of coffee, the instant
> variety.
>
> (Fieldnotes, Normans' Funeral Parlour)

Funeral parlours tend to use 'olde worlde' furniture and trimmings. This comforting air of stability and conventionality can easily slide into a feeling of staleness. Margaret found her funeral director's office 'seedy'; I know what she means.

An expression of 'traditional values' is to be found in the current fashion of offering horse-drawn funerals. The Victorian funeral is held up as an emblem of the golden past of death: not surprising when we consider that this extravagant period saw the birth of this very industry (Curl 1972). Another theme, that of social mobility through conspicuous consumption at death, is also still apparent.

> I have my tyres boot-polished. Everything is impeccable. The standard is as good as anything that comes out of the Royal Mews. And that's the standard that we retain.
>
> (Mr Black, Black's Funeral Parlour)

There are signs of change within the industry as a new generation of customers come in to arrange their elderly relative's funerals. Some of the more innovative firms have revamped their image, rejecting the old black suit and somewhat sombre parlour interiors in favour of more informal outfits and tastefully decorated rooms that feel more like a fashionable dentist's surgery. These changes have caused some consternation in the more traditional family-run firms.

> He has got those blinking grey suits, company ties, girls looking like hostesses, you know, with the scarves around their neck . . . And they have got all this business of showing them photographs [of coffins], you know, and selling. Pushing.
>
> (Mr Black, Black's Funeral Parlour)

A central and important figure in the funeral industry is the funeral director. They liaise with mortuaries, clergy, cemeteries, crematoria and florists on behalf of the bereaved client who usually contact them the day after a death. I was struck by the generally glowing accounts of the funeral director. These descriptions of thoughtful, kind and helpful service seemed at odds with media descriptions of an industry that is ripping us off. My findings seem to mirror those of Fulton (1965), working in America, who found that the public were generally not critical of funeral directors. It seems very possible that people simply accept the fact that the kindness of the funeral director is in part motivated by commerce.

I think Rogers' were, in fact, quite excellent. They were
thoroughly supportive and very helpful.

(Susan)

Funeral parlours rarely advertise. As one funeral director admitted,
'We are the advertising man's nightmare, selling something no one
wants to buy.' There seems little evidence that people conduct much
market research before choosing a funeral parlour. The widows I
interviewed either relied on recommendations or picked the nearest
high street firm. Not one of my informants rang two or more funeral
parlours to compare services or prices. Most people will only arrange
one or two funerals in their lives which means that the majority of us
are not funereal experts. While funeral directors must be aware that
they may not see this particular client again, a good funeral parlour
does make a name for itself in the community.

You may imagine that funeral directors set their fees as they think
fit. This is a popular media accusation. Yet allegations of the exploit-
ation of the bereaved do not really stand up to scrutiny. Although
funerals are expensive, costing well over £1000 in London, they are
not overpriced when we take into account the high costs of labour and
the huge overheads involved in running a funeral business. Each shiny
black hearse and limousine, for example, costs more than £50,000.
Similarly, it is commonly supposed that funeral directors employ
hard-sell techniques (Mitford 1963). While this may be the case in
some rare instances, it would generally be an unwise move on the part
of the undertakers. They have to pay for the costs of the burial or
cremation before they receive payment from the bereaved, so it is not
in their interest to make people overextend themselves. Every parlour
has plenty of experience of bad debts.

I am aware that I sound as if I have been sold over to the undertakers
trade, but, as Richardson (personal communication) has noted, it is
perfectly possible that this trade is the victim of scapegoating. Our
negative representation of the business of undertaking may be a
reflection of our fears about death.

The interview at the parlour

The plan of a funeral parlour demonstrates a split between front and
back of house. The front – public rooms consist of a reception,
waiting-room, interviewing-rooms and viewing chapel while backstage, out of bounds, we find the workshop, storeroom, refrigeration
and embalming-room, garages and general office. Howarth (1996), in

a detailed study of funeral directing, notes how the body gradually works its way forward from the private to the public spaces of the parlour, with increasing ceremony as it goes forward. This reaches a peak in the funeral parlour's viewing chapel, a place where the body and the bereaved come together in one of their rare meetings. Parlours are designed to give an air of privacy, if not secrecy. Waiting and interview rooms are often much like cubicles, either windowless, or with heavily curtained or frosted glass.

Although undertakers will come to a person's house to make the arrangements, most people visit them at their shop. There are more forms to sign and more questions to answer. Like the registrar and the coroner, the besuited funeral director often sits behind an imposing desk, looking for all the world like a bank manager. Prior notes how 'they are keen to be perceived as professionals and often pin certificates of competence and qualification on the walls of their offices, much as an optician, a dental surgeon or a pharmacist might do' (1989: 160). During my visits to parlours, I was struck by how often my attention was directed to these certificates by proud directors.

> I sat in on an interview with a woman who had just lost her young son. She was accompanied by an elderly male friend of hers. I sat on a chair by one side, in the tiny office. Typically, this office was bare except for a calendar, a desk, a few chairs and some cheap prints. The funeral director was quite clever at posing his questions, alternating between the easy, 'What's your name?', and the more difficult, 'And what would you like Andrew to be wearing?' However, she was clearly stumped by his question about clothes and burst into tears.
>
> (Fieldnotes, Dent's Funeral Parlour)

> When we are talking about the viewing, and the coffin . . . usually that goes with the interior or the coffin and the gown set. Umm, so it would be a question more on the lines of, you know, 'Unless you had any particular wishes, we will dress your mother, or father, just in an ordinary funeral gown.' And just see what the response is. Nine times out of ten it is just 'Right, that will be fine.'
>
> (Funeral Director, Dent's Funeral Homes)

The meeting with the funeral director is at least the third interview the bereaved will have had in the course of the past 24 hours and marks an important moment in the passage of the bereaved through the social organization of death. It is at this point that decisions are made about the disposal of the body. The bereaved client has to commit themselves to a certain number of poignant decisions during this interview: what will the deceased wear?; what kind of coffin would the deceased have preferred?; are they going to have their loved one cremated or buried? Answering these questions can have a strong effect on people. Directors are aware of this and tiptoe through the minefield, carefully and skilfully extracting the information they need without causing too many emotional outbursts. They often have to keep an eye on the clock.

It is only when things don't go according to plan that you get tensed up. Because of the way that I am. And because of the fact that whatever happens the family shouldn't see it. Then everything tends to happen inside me. If I am arranging a funeral and I am due out at another funeral in ten minutes time, and I know that this is going to take a quarter of an hour, all I can think is that I am going to be five minutes late, getting inwardly tense.

(Funeral Director, Haynes' Funeral Homes)

Arranging a date is a tricky operation for the funeral director as many London crematoria and cemeteries are booked-up for a week or more in advance. A booking on the day the family hoped for may simply not be possible. Directors leave the room to make their phone calls to the local 'crems' and 'cems', as crematoria and cemeteries are known in the trade. Meanwhile the family will have been left to collect themselves. This can also be an opportunity for the bereaved to flick through the albums of glossy photographs of coffins and caskets, although some directors like to keep these out of sight.

You then have to sit and look at the book of coffins. To decide which one you want. I mean, looking back on it I think, if that had been today, I would have probably thrown it at them. But you don't, you accept all this, just sitting there, you know.

(Paula)

I remember my daughter saying 'Oh, for goodness sake, I do hope he doesn't bring a brochure!' Like a Habitat catalogue. And sure enough, he produced the brochure. So we went into peals of laughter, I think he thought we were batty.

(Eleanor)

Deathwork: picking up the body

The next task for the funeral director is to pick up the corpse from the hospital mortuary or the family home. During the interview with the bereaved, the funeral director is unlikely to talk about how and when they will collect the corpse from the mortuary; such details are not deemed relevant. The funeral director's access to the hospital mortuary, usually discretely positioned in the back or basement of hospital buildings, is confined to certain opening hours, in which funeral parlours can collect the dead. Usually, undertakers use unmarked, often white, vans for this pick-up run although if things are very busy the body may be carried in the lower section of a hearse: still conspicuous but at least the body is hidden from view. This is a time when the death is not being advertised.

Many funeral firms now offer a 24-hour service. This is often emphasized in their advertisements in the Yellow Pages. Although it costs more to remove a body from the home in the middle of the night, the very fact that the service is on offer creates a felt need to get the body out of the house and reflects expectations that such behaviour is seemly. If people do express a wish to retain the body at home, then they would find that most funeral directors would apply subtle pressure to have the body removed and embalmed first.

Just as the terminal support team have to find a way of creating a backstage when working with a dying person at home, undertakers who arrive at a private address in order to remove the body are keen to work away from the eyes of watching relatives. They argue that putting a body into a body bag and strapping it on to a trolley is a disturbing and physical act which relatives should not witness.

> But they have to strap them up. But I said 'Why do you wrap him up like a parcel?' and one of them turned to me and said 'You don't want him to fall out when we get him through the door do you?' I was a fool to myself. I knew they had to move him, and I could see that the straps stopped him from falling through the door. They have this funny trolley with two wheels. I was a fool to myself. Janet [the terminal support nurse] had told me to stay in the bedroom, but I'd said I wanted to stay.
>
> (Christine)

Members of the family are usually urged to wait in another room. There is an ever-present risk of disease. Officially, funeral staff are supposed to wear full protective clothes, including face masks, whenever they pick up a body from home. I was told by the funeral director at Dent's that this makes him feel silly – turning up in all that gear while the family are dressed as usual. He only does so if the GP has warned him beforehand of the risks of, say, contracting TB or becoming infected with the HIV virus.

Deathwork: embalming

Went into the embalming-room. He opened the door and I saw two naked corpses, sprawled on their trollies. Uncovered. In the cold. The director turned to me and said 'Have you seen bodies before?' Well, yes and no. I said yes and that I appreciated him asking. In we went. I was very relieved when he steered me to another end of the room, past the bank of refrigerators, past the blackboard with the dead people's names on it. Back into the embalmer's room. Let's meet the embalmer. Carefully steered out of sight of the bodies. He peels off a rubber glove, I swallow and shake his hand. I guess he appreciates my handshake. I inch into the view of the dead. The two old people with their backsides in view and their white feet and skinny legs have been covered with a piece of paper. They still look vulnerable and exposed.

Then, with something of a jolt, I realize that round the corner, out of sight, lie a whole row of the dead. About seven corpses lined up. Some dressed. Some half-dressed. Some embalmed. I gaze and gaze. I see one of the old ladies has a black toe and suddenly I'm gone; I'm going to faint. Now it's a struggle. I can feel the blood drain from my face and I have lost the sense of feeling in my lips. My head is whirring. I keep talking and I'm still making sense. But I know that I'm now in shock.

I look again. One sixty-something dad, fully embalmed, wearing his acrylic Saturday jumper. The tattoo on his plumped-up embalmed arm. He looks good, I have to say. The beautiful dead. All lined up. All peaceful. Very quiet. I think that one of them is breathing, but I guess that I'm now on the wild side. Hallucinating. It doesn't smell so good. Old refrigerated chicken. The embalming room is very cool.

We leave. I am stunned to find myself continuing my calm performance. Out of the room and back to the office. I sit down. I take some deep breaths. Somewhere it is fine. Thanks Ethel, thanks William – and all the others.

(Fieldnotes, Brown's Funeral Parlour)

Back in the parlour, bodies are usually refrigerated at first. Embalming is usually carried out a couple of days later. The contents of the lower colon, the centre of decomposition, are suctioned and replaced by sterilizing fluid. The blood is also replaced with embalming fluid (formaldehyde and pink dye) which is added to the arteries while the blood is either drained from the veins if the body is fresh or suctioned out of the body cavity if the corpse is a few days old. If necessary, false teeth are inserted. The mouth is then sewn shut. The eyeballs are covered by domed plastic over which the lids are stuck. A man will have a shave or his beard or moustache will be trimmed. The hair is dressed and powder and make-up may be applied to the face and hands. In the extract that follows I grapple with the shock of seeing a corpse being embalmed.

Brian offers to show me an embalming. First, he proudly demonstrates the difference between embalmed and non-embalmed corpses. Two ninety-year-old ladies. One embalmed, the other in something of a bad way after a post-mortem (brain and organs removed, bad staining of her skin). I don't feel as awful as I did last time, strangely. Not faint. Just kind of nervous and jumpy. I keep fidgeting.

Brian then wheels the gent he is about to embalm into position. First he breaks up the rigor mortis. I am not sure how much I want to see. Then Brian shows me how he gets out the artery from the armpit region into which he will be pumping the formaldehyde. It is a bit grim, watching him digging around. The old man's arm keeps waving around, stiffly embracing Brian's waist. The corpse seems to be trying to stop him. I gaze at this old man's body laid out under the bright lights. His fine handsome face. A military man, by the looks of him. Cotton wool has been plugged into his mouth and I worry that he cannot breathe or will gag.

Meanwhile, Brian has now started pumping in the embalming fluid. The hand changes quite dramatically. I am really surprised by the change. Gone the really blue look, replaced by a kind of pinky yellow look. The hand and then the face look quite a lot better. Oh, embalming is not so bad. I go for a little explore elsewhere, have a look at the refrigerators and the storeroom filled with coffins of every size, which is kind of touching (in an odd sort of way). Every now and then I peep at what Brian is doing. For the benefit of my research. The hole under the arm is sutured. I hope he has sterilized the needle; oh, it doesn't matter, does it?

Next time I look Brian is working on removing the blood.

Using a long-handled hollow probe which is manipulated around the body cavity. He is 'breaking down' the organs. This is ugly work. I suddenly don't feel so good about embalming. The work looks unpleasant and a bit shocking. It is somehow strangely distressing to see the old man being pushed around in this way. He needs those organs, doesn't he?

Nails are scrubbed and cleaned. A shave, a trim of the moustache. False teeth added, the mouth sewn shut with stitches through the bottom gum and out through the nostrils; ugh.

(Fieldnotes, Brown's Funeral Parlour)

Great care is made to hide any suture marks from a post-mortem and, if the person died as a result of a disfiguring accident, the embalmer will sew up wounds and suture on an amputated limb, etc. When presenting the body in the coffin, hair and clothing are used to hide any scars. While the end product may look and smell a lot better than it did beforehand, in truth it is likely to look very different from the familiar and living vision of that beloved person. From the perspective of the bereaved, the make-up, the unfamiliar hairstyle and the slightly fat and pink face just make the corpse look more embalmed than anything else.

Viewing at the parlour

She showed me the viewing room. Awful. Yet another tiny, windowless room. Thick carpets and a terrible smell of dust and embalming preservative. There were two curtained sections, behind which the coffins are placed on a niche in the wall. The place was very dimly lit. I found this room incredibly spooky and would have hated to have viewed in such a place. All red decor and no air.

(Fieldnotes, Molesworth's Funeral Parlour)

Most funeral directors recommend viewing unless the body is badly disfigured. People usually come to view three or four days after the death. The open coffin is set up in the viewing chapel before the family's arrival. Viewing is a highly charged moment for the bereaved family. During the preceeding few days, the body has changed a great deal as the result of decomposition, embalming, make-up and possibly unusual clothing. In the last few days the body has travelled along a very different path from that of those who survived it and the palpable distance between the living and the dead is now dramatically obvious.

This is the moment when the relatives are likely to be forcibly struck by the finality of death.

> He [the funeral director] showed me around his parlour. Walked, with some trepidation, towards the viewing rooms. Shown in. First chapel had just a coffin. That was bad enough. Behind that closed lid lay a body. Next room, horrors of horrors, an open coffin. A body. A nice old man. Very thin, very old. I felt quite shocked. But he was kind of calming. I noticed that I kept imagining that his chest was rising and falling. He was very pale and very, well, dead.
>
> Next chapel room. Another old lady. She had fallen. I kept my distance. Her name was Daisy. She was very old. She had a bruise on her chin. A fall. I got closer and looked at the bruise. The embalming job was good, not too much make-up. Next chapel room. Another grandma, once again covered with a fly cover with lacy trim. I looked at her plumped-up lips. She still looked very, very dead. But once again I thought I saw her chest rising and falling. My own heart was pounding.
>
> (Fieldnotes, Brown's Funeral Parlour)

Funeral directors are aware of the traumatic nature of this meeting and nowhere are their subtle skills in manipulating emotions more in demand. One funeral director said he briefed people beforehand, telling them that the deceased 'looks wonderful' so that they would feel satisfied with the embalming efforts, however much of a shock. He quaintly described this as 'directing their expectations upwards'. Apparently, there are huge variations in the amount of time that people want to spend viewing. Some people literally walk in and out, others wish to spend many hours with the body. One parlour I visited had decided to build a second, long-stay viewing chapel to cater for the second type of viewer.

The 'wait'

Having viewed the body the relatives normally have to wait a few days until their 'slot' at the cemetery or crematorium comes round. This can be a harrowing time. Many of my respondents found the wait difficult as, on the one hand, they dreaded the day of the funeral yet, on the other, they found the fact that the deceased was not yet laid to rest distressing. During the winter months the wait can be extended to two weeks or more as cemeteries and crematoria struggle with the increased death rates caused by influenza epidemics and such like. During this time the relatives face the funeral-related tasks of planning the service, ordering flowers and liaising with people who will be coming on the day. After this respite comes more activity and more contact with the professionals.

A common misconception among the recently bereaved is that the cemetery or the crematorium plays a role similar to that of the funeral director: namely that they will arrange a funeral. Regularly, confused relatives telephone their local cemetery or crematorium just after the death. They are redirected to the undertaker. As one cemetery manager succinctly put it, 'The bereaved are nothing to do with me, that's the funeral director's job.' Indeed, most crematoria and cemeteries will only deal with those funerals arranged by a funeral director. This practice is increasingly coming under pressure from social innovators who argue that the bereaved family are entitled to arrange their own funeral without the funeral director's help if they so wish.

The funeral cortège

The passage of the coffin from the funeral parlour or the home to its final place of rest has always been seen as a very significant event, although its meaning has changed over the years. Before the industrial revolution, carrying the coffin from the home to the churchyard had been a moment when the whole community was made aware of the death. During this passage the family, walking or in carriages, prepared themselves for the first and final separation. In the Victorian era the cortège still set off from the home, but the message to the community was somewhat different. Rather than merely informing the local community in order to allow them to pay their last respects, the Victorian cortège expressed the wealth of the deceased. The modern day cortège is a descendant of the Victorian one and the message it conveys of conspicuous consumption is still important to some. I was told of East End funerals in which the hearse was followed by ten limousines. However, for the majority of mourners, following the coffin is merely something that the funeral director suggested. Nowadays, the coffin does not set off from the home, but from the funeral parlour. The hearse is driven to the home where the relatives are picked up. Thus, instead of parting from the coffin, the relatives often see the coffin for the first time in its glass display in the hearse. The meaning has been reversed. Rather than being a passage in which the relatives prepare to separate, it is a meeting point in which the relatives try to cope with the shock of the changed appearance of the body, now encased in a coffin and covered in the flowers the relatives had carefully chosen a few days before.

After this short, ceremonial trip, the mourners and the deceased arrive at the crematorium or cemetery. Having unloaded the coffin and flowers and having seated the guests inside the chapel or church, the funeral director seems to lose interest in the proceedings. For many undertakers, the service is of little interest. Normally funeral directors and drivers hang around outside, smoking or chatting, while the clergy 'do their bit'. Meanwhile the empty hearse is sent off to pick up another coffin for the next funeral.

Burial and cremation

The acts of cremation and of burial are very different. In burial the coffins are placed in single, shared or common graves. Most graves are not owned in perpetuity, which in fact means 100 years, but are rented for a fixed number of years. Most leases last for 50 years or so. The land can then be recycled. However, the urban cemeteries in and around London are either full or soon will be and there are not enough grave spaces ready for recycling. Discussions are currently being held for the implementation of the rapid recycling of graves at 20 or 25 years with disinterment followed by either the cremation of any remains found or the reburial of remains at a deeper level (called 'lift and rebury'). On the Continent, remains are removed to a bone ossary on site.

Cremation is currently the more popular form of disposal. In cremation the body is incinerated by furnaces specially designed for the task. Cremation creates a secondary product: ashes. The public appear to be mystified by the nature of ashes. What, exactly, is in them? Are they really the ashes of your loved one, or does the crematorium hand over just anyone's? The high temperatures involved in cremation mean that only the bones and the metal pins, bolts and staples from the coffin are left. These metal products are later removed by an electro-magnet. Most of the wood goes up the chimney. Crematoria make strenuous efforts to retain the integrity or individuality of each person's remains. There is no crude mixing of ashes. Sensitive to people's ambivalent feelings towards ashes, most crematoria offer a 'holding service' whereby the ashes are stored at the crematorium, for a small rental fee, while the bereaved decide what to do with them. Ashes can be placed in a columbarium or scattered in some favourite site or on top of an old family gravesite in the local cemetery. They may also be interred underground.

Recently, Jupp (1993) investigated people's reasons for choosing either cremation or burial. He found that people made decisions concerning disposal on the basis of their social identity (e.g. socio-economic background and religion) and the mundane but nevertheless powerful motive of convenience. Cremation is certainly cheaper than burial in London, although some crematorium memorials can cost as much as a grave. For cemeteries the major costs arise from the purchase or reopening of a grave. Purchasing a new grave in a London borough costs more than £1000.00, while moving the headstone of a previously purchased grave can easily run into several hundred pounds. A new headstone can cost £1000.00.

Because of the large amount of land these institutions require, both crematoria and cemeteries tend to be sited at the edge of the city. I visited several crematoria and cemeteries. I noted a certain difference between those owned by the borough and those owned by private companies. The former had a local council parks feel, while the latter tended to be a little more luxurious. Nevertheless, publicly or privately owned, profit is a motive that lies behind both types.

> It is profit-making, not subsidized. You see, at £90.00 a cremation and 4500 a year. It usually pays for itself.
>
> (Manager, borough crematorium)

It is the funeral director's task to make sure the certificate for disposal and the cremation forms get to the administration office at the crematorium at least the day before the funeral. The crematorium is duty bound to make yet another doctor, often working in occupational health, scan the cremation form to check that they are satisfied that the cause of death described in forms B and C are clear. Within the industry, the use of the third medical referee is often viewed as a totally superfluous and outdated activity. Everyone acknowledges that the choice of cause of death was a form of intelligent guesswork and it is rare for the second doctor to contradict the doctor who met the deceased while terminally ill. It is even rarer for the crematorium's doctor to query a pair of certificates, although this does happen occasionally.

Like the hospital and funeral parlour, these sites are clearly split into front and backstage areas. The frontstage section is made up of car-park, reception rooms and chapels; the backstage section of general cremators, offices and staff rooms. This extract is from my fieldnotes after a visit to a private crematorium.

I was then shown the 'behind the scenes' section. The change from the chapel and waiting-rooms was striking. The public space had been chapelesque in its nature, formal and old fashioned. Behind the doors I got the feeling that I had entered a hospital ward. White walls and tiled floors replaced terracotta and wood. The coffin was dragged on to a hospital body trolley and pushed into the waiting area in front of the row of cremators. In a somewhat dramatic way, the attendant told me that once the body had passed through the swing doors to this space, it couldn't be removed unless there was a court injunction to do so.

Walking through another set of swing doors, I came across the 'furnace' doors, manned by four cremator operators, who made sure that oxygen levels and temperatures were right and that rakings were carried out. This area felt rather like a ship's stoking-room. The heat and smell of burning were very noticeable. I was taken into a small office room adjoining the furnace room. One of the operators ghoulishly showed me all the oddities collected from the rakings over the years: old-fashioned bone-pins, artificial hips and the like. There were drawers of them. He then showed me the books that he had to fill in, making a big point about the way he never got the ashes mixed up. He then asked me if I would like to see a body burn. I was horrified, yet tried to hide it. Said I really didn't think it would help my research.

Finally I was shown another little room where the ashes are ground up by a machine. On shelves above are lined rows upon rows of plastic containers, each carefully labelled, full of grey ashes. It felt just like a potting shed.

(Fieldnotes, private crematorium)

The committal service

Observing a funeral . . . This was a place of regimental gravestones. There was a lot of mud around, as the graves had been dug by machine. The mourners really did look wretched as the coffin was lowered; some were crying. The priest said a few words, before some of the mourners threw in some earth. Then they drifted away – it couldn't have taken longer than ten minutes. This surprised me.

(Fieldnotes, borough cemetery)

The committal occurs when the body is put in the grave, the crematorium furnace or the sea. This is not always the end of the story, however. For example, graves are often reopened and released to make room for other occupants. The committal service in burial is relatively clear-cut although it does take place in two stages. In front of the mourners the body is lowered into the ground and soil is ceremonially thrown on top of the coffin. Later, once the mourners have gone home, the grave will be fully covered with soil by the grave-diggers.

In cremation, this drawing out of the committal service is more exaggerated. First, there is a pseudo-committal when the coffin is either trundled out of sight, lowered to a basement level, left in place or, most frequently, covered by a curtain in the chapel of the crematorium (Davies 1997). Later, backstage, the first real committal occurs when the coffin is put into the furnace. With the exception of British Hindus, whose chief mourners may either help to push the coffin into the cremator or will observe the coffin being automatically pushed into the cremator, it is rare for the general public to enter this backstage space. Watching the coffin disappear behind the curtain can be something of a ritual non-event. Everyone knows that this first, public, cremation committal is false. The coffin and corpse are still whole, lying in another room or hidden by a curtain. Quite naturally, the bereaved wonder what will happen backstage. Will the attendants recycle the coffin? Will they tear off the fake-brass fittings? Is the body cremated today or tomorrow? At a potentially significant moment the participants are cast into doubt and confusion. Indeed, such fears of malpractice seem to be a dim and distant echo of eighteenth- and nineteenth-century obsessions with outwitting the resurrectionists.

People often talk of the cremation service as being 'like a conveyor belt'. In an analysis of this metaphor, D. J. Davies (1996) notes that unlike traditional churches, in which participants use the same door to enter and exit, most crematoria chapels have a main door for entry and a side door for exit. It is the presence of the next funeral party waiting at the main door and the sense of being part of a flow of participants which, he argues, engenders that feeling of being 'processed'. In this instance, a convenient flow of people through an architectural space has not necessarily been a successful innovation. Davies suggests that, over time, the concept of the participants moving away from the coffin, which remains behind the curtain, could be viewed as an appropriate part of the process of mourning and disposing: a statement of change.

Aspects of belief

This is a multicultural society and it would take another book to describe the great variety of religious practice at the time of a death (see Laungani and Morgan 1998). As my research subjects were all Christian I have limited myself to a discussion of broadly Christian ideals.

> The service where everyone believes, they see death as a continuation, and that what he is going to is better than what he is leaving. It's a joyful thing, a celebration. Tears and happiness go together.
>
> (The Reverend John Jones)

> The funeral was absolutely beautiful. We had all the most wonderful music, and the church was full, and that was very comforting.
>
> (Beth)

Many Church of England clergymen and women regularly find themselves playing an important, if not central, part in the funeral. Religious funerals can truly be a celebration of a life well lived and of a future of eternal peace. In such instances, the vicar will visit the family and offer much-needed support and consolation. Focusing on the positive impact of attending funerals, Davies (1997) argues that funeral rites offer the participants an opportunity of gaining a heightened sense of identity and purpose through participation in them. He emphasizes the strong verbal component in rituals, arguing that these 'performance utterances' (1997: 7) can have extraordinary power or force. The committal service can be seen as the moment at which the deceased meets their maker and the bereaved are faced with the truth of mortality; in the process the participants are transformed. On the basis of my research it was obvious that there are still mortuary rites that operate on these higher levels and participation in these funerals can be 'life enhancing'. Months after the event, the sacred feelings evoked by the service were vividly remembered.

There have always been varying degrees of religiosity, and for those who have not exactly lived their lives in the arms of the established church, death can be a time when religious belief and practice is gratefully leaned on. Even for those who do not belong to any kind of religious institution and for whom the afterlife remains a very hazy concept, a good religious send-off with a few familiar hymns can still seem a natural choice. If the family do not know whom to choose to officiate at the funeral they very often turn to the funeral director for help. If people belonging nominally to the Church of England are not known to their local vicar, the funeral director is expected to inform the local vicar that a member of their parish has died. Indeed, Canon 'B38' dictates that it is the 'duty' of all Anglican clergy 'to bury, according to the rites of the Church of England, the corpse or ashes of any person deceased within his cure or of any parishioner or persons whose names are entered on the church electoral role of his parish . . . ' However, the custom of funeral directors letting vicars know of local deaths is not formalized, so many funeral directors do not bother. It is tedious for them to deal with clergymen and women from many different parishes and the last thing a funeral director wants is a busy clergyman or woman who is not able to make appointments because of other commitments. Instead, many funeral directors turn to their 'tame' clergyman who can be relied on to be flexible about times.

There are also a great many people who are either atheist or agnostic. For these people, traditional rituals officiated by a clergyman or woman may simply fail to make sense. Lacking belief and adopting a passive role in the proceedings, it is easy for such people to observe the funeral as an outsider and to feel that it is merely arbitrary or conventional (Hockey 1990). Such participants see the underbelly of our rituals: that apparently desperate effort to deny that death is the end. It is little wonder that contemporary funerals are then accused by these people of being empty or hollow. We do not have to have a religious funeral and there are other options. Nevertheless I found that very few funeral directors informed their clients that they are perfectly entitled to conduct their own humanist or rationalist committal ceremony. Concerned that a DIY committal service would run over-time, the directors felt happier in suggesting to their clients that they use a good clergyman who would do the job for them without too much talk of God. In such instances when people without faith find themselves attending a semi-religious service conducted by a stranger, the participants face not just the loss of their loved one but may also the loss of meaning itself (Hockey 1990).

Hockey (1993) highlighted the ways in which clergy visualized the emotion of grief. On the basis of interviews Hockey revealed that the clergy officiating over funeral services worked on the widespread Western model of emotion in which grief was viewed as a natural and uncontrollable entity, a kind of natural force contained within the body, ready to spring. She notes that such a view of emotion, in which we presume it is desirable to release these pent-up feelings, is in conflict with the religious official's desire to conduct the rather structured committal service. Thus she found clergy were embroiled in a delicate balancing act in which they struggled with the contradiction between encouraging the expression of emotions and the desire to sustain an orderly service. I found funeral directors, who increasingly are coming to see themselves in therapeutic terms, were also engaged in such a precarious balancing act.

In our secular society there are signs that the clergy's traditional role is changing. Given the stark contrast between the funeral services of those families who know their vicar and who have faith, and those who find themselves attending a funeral conducted by someone they do not know and do not believe in, we can understand why members of the clergy have doubts about the suitability of officiating over all funerals. One clergyman mentioned that, when asked to preside over agnostic or atheist funerals, he felt constrained to alter the focus of his sermon. Rather than talk of the sense of celebration and resignation at death he felt his secular audience would only be interested in talk of sadness and sorrow at their loss. Recently, efforts have been made to address these issues (see General Synod debate 1998, Special Agenda IV, Item 802). It is clear that the clergy's role in our death practices will continue to be debated for some time.

Commerce versus ritual

Most funeral directors have a 'tame' or 'pet' clergyman, as they are referred to, who is called in whenever there is a need. A tame clergyman is a vicar, often retired, who is willing to do any date offered to him. Many funeral directors do not want to juggle the schedules of client, crematorium or cemetery with those of a vicar. Indeed, during the busy winter months such negotiations may be impossible. When a tame clergyman is employed, the vicar will not know the family and he may not even visit them, although most do. There are, after all, clear guidelines available to all clergy, even tame ones (see *Guidelines for Best Practice of Clergy at Funerals*, published by The Churches' Group in 1997 and *In Sure and Certain Hope: Best Funeral Practice*, Diocese of Norwich). Working with the larger funeral companies a tame clergyman could spend his whole day at the local crematorium, earning approximately £70.00 for each service.

Mr Black, a funeral director with strong opinions, believed that another important characteristic of the tame clergyman was that he would not 'sell God'. In this instance it is absolutely clear that the perceived role of the clergy is not so much religious as palliative. This seems to finds echoes in Hockey's (1993) findings, discussed above. Mr Black's 'man' from the Baptist church down the road was taken 'everywhere I go'. He kept things short and didn't waste everybody's time with talk of heaven.

> I always go round and I listen. While [the minister is] talking. And one thing I listen [to] in particular [is] the way the service is conducted. I listen out for that . . . Because I keep, basically, one man who does most of mine. Because of the way he does it . . . [I am] disappointed and disillusioned with some of the clergy because of their attitude . . . You know, they will get out The Book and dar de dar de dar . . . There is a time and a place for all that. All right if they were a religious type of family, you know, communicants and regular churchgoers. [But] there is not many of them about, let's be honest.
>
> (Mr Black, Black's Funeral Parlour)

Maybe the rather unrealistic clergyman needs to be matched by the pragmatic undertaker! Who has got his eye on the watch thinking, 'Well, I hope he'll finish soon because we have the next one in three minutes.' Because, you see, it is terrible, particularly in London crematoria, where, as you probably know, twenty minutes and the next lot are queuing up and it's all got to be done as smoothly as possible. I think [the funeral director] really has got to be master of ceremonies, in a way.

> (The Reverend Ralph Peters)

Historically, the relationship between funeral directors and the clergy has never been an easy one. There is always a tension between the perceived importance of roles of these two very different sets of people. Fulton, in a study conducted with members of the clergy in the early 1960s found that 'clerical criticism of the funeral director and of funeral practices was both widespread and intense' (Fulton 1995: 193). He uncovered two main complaints: the funeral director's tendency to ignore the spiritual aspects of death and the director's ability to take advantage of the bereaved. I found that criticisms from funeral directors against the clergy were healthily balanced by the disdain and criticism levelled at them by the clergy who often viewed them as businessmen. This mild state of war is undeclared.

> I have got one or two friends who are funeral directors, so they are not all bad. But I think they are motivated largely by expediency,

and well, convenience and . . . they are busy. And also, some of them are not terribly, or the people who work with them, this sounds terribly snobbish, but they are not terribly aware, or, sophisticated.

(The Reverend Ralph Peters)

Waking the dead

It was absolutely a gorgeous day. And they had all salads and things, which is rather nice. And, again, I must have thought I was at some sort of reception, because I kept doing this 'You all right?', 'Got plenty to eat?', 'Sure you won't have a drink?' You know, gadding around.

(Paula)

I just went upstairs. I knew that this room would be too full. I never came down, I was upstairs. So people would come looking for me.

(Kate)

The committal service is usually followed by some kind of wake. Normally this takes place at the home of the deceased. Family and friends make up most of the visitors, although others, such as funeral directors, clergy, work colleagues and neighbours are often also invited. Refreshments are served. Invariably friends and family take over the task of preparing the food. In the past wakes preceded the committal and the party centred around the encoffined corpse. In the absence of the deceased, modern day wakes, occurring after the funeral, often seem to lack such a focus. Ruth unobtrusively lit a candle to represent her husband's presence in their crowded sitting room.

I lit a candle for my husband. So that he was present. I still have the candle. It was nice, because it was all among the people.

(Ruth)

Remembering the dead

We got his name in the book of remembrance. I went yesterday. I mean, I don't go and sit and cry or anything. You know. But I like to sit in the chapel for a little while.

(Doris)

Apart from the day of the funeral, the only personal contact the public is likely to have with the crematorium or cemetery occurs when they come to purchase the memorials. Both borough and private cemeteries and crematoria offer memorials for sale, although the marketing in the private firms seems to be more aggressive. Salespeople are sometimes called 'memorial counsellors', which says a great deal about our therapy-orientated culture. I found that members of the funeral trade have been keen to capitalize on lay models of psychological research which suggest that a healthy grief reaction is one in which the bereaved face the reality of death. Within the trade this has been reinterpreted as making the most of the various funerary artefacts on sale.

Cemetery memorials are relatively uniform. In contrast to the eccentric headstones and statues which were popular 100 years ago, contemporary headstones are controlled by cemetery regulations which dictate height, material, shape and wording, etc. Generally, however, efforts are made to accommodate people's desires in memorialization, unless they are too outlandish. People can also purchase benches and, on occasion, trees and shrubs.

Most crematoria offer a wide selection of memorials, many of which are similar to those on sale at a cemetery, while some are a little more unusual. Most crematoria (and a few cemeteries) have a chapel of remembrance, which houses the 'book of remembrance'. The book of remembrance is a large leather book, in appearance much like a Bible. Each day it is opened at the appropriate page, displaying the details of the death anniversaries. Mourners purchase entries in these books of remembrance and each hand-written entry has the name, date of birth, date of death, plus sentimental and personal comment. Occasionally, these epitaphs are a challenge to good taste and in such instances, staff are faced with the delicate task of negotiation with the grieving client. For an extra fee, the entry can be illustrated with flowers, scrolls or crests. This book is placed under a glass cover in a prominent place in the chapel. Tiny 'booklets of remembrance', which contain a copy of the original entry, are also on sale. I was told these make a great gift.

The chapel may offer other opportunities for capitalistic gain or for sentimental expression, depending on your point of view. You can buy or rent wall plaques and candle or plant holders (which grace the walls of the chapel). You can see how it would be easy to spend hundreds of pounds on these objects. Although this kind of marketing can make us feel somewhat cynical, it does seem to serve a purpose. I was quite impressed by the atmosphere created by these floral, verbal and architectural tributes.

In the extracts that follow we can note the difference between the borough crematoria and the private crematoria.

The chapel of remembrance was a cold room, which had recently been built. In the centre was placed the book of remembrance, put under glass. The room didn't feel like a chapel at all, more like a conservatory, if anything. There was also a small garden of remembrance. The beds were white with what appeared to be strewn ashes. Apparently, the garden was so small there were no facilities for renting rose bushes, etc.

(Fieldnotes, borough crematorium)

The memorial chapel was packed with flowers, which people had brought in and left in the stands made available for this purpose. Others had bought, or rented, wallspaces, in which candles and flowers are held. The place smelt wonderful. The book of remembrance was given pride of place, opened at the appropriate place for the particular day. I was quite surprised to see the number of people sitting quietly in this chapel: there must have been at least a dozen. I then walked into the memorial gardens. Well-designed, but absolutely overflowing with memorial plaques, urns, rose-bushes and what-not. The main lawn was covered with memorial crocuses, which the bereaved could purchase for a few pounds. Ashes were sprinkled on this lawn, or buried (for a rented rate) under rose bushes, trees, etc. The garden was actually quite pleasant to walk through.

(Fieldnotes, private crematorium)

As I mentioned previously, cremation takes place 'backstage' in an object – the cremator – that is both communal and functional. During cremation and the storage of the ashes prior to their final disposal, the remains of the deceased are not located at a site at which the survivors may mourn. On the one hand, this may explain why crematoria offer a wide and eclectic selection of memorials, such as books and poems, which are not necessarily geographically bound. On the other hand, the promiscuous character of the cremator and the potentially vagrant nature of the remains may be precisely what causes such efforts to put the ashes in one final, personal resting place.

The importance of mortuary practices in anchoring the dead has been noted in non-industrial groups (Bloch 1971). A burial gives the mourners a site at which they can collect to remember and grieve. It is possible that the choice of British burial memorials reflects this situational anchoring of grief in times when many families are geographically dispersed, for many memorials are weighty and solid.

We can therefore see that the cremation of the dead poses some dilemmas to the survivors. Each corpse is cremated in a cremator which is used by many other corpses. The cremator itself does not offer any opportunity for personal memorialization. Indeed, for many it is an object of some horror, conjuring up images of the holocaust (Davies 1997). In contrast, the resulting ashes are portable and can be taken anywhere. Usually, great effort is put into anchoring these homeless remains, whether this is done inside the crematorium walls or at some private, sentimental site. You can purchase or plant memorial flowers, bulbs, bushes or trees. The mourners can further consolidate their, admittedly tenuous, ownership of the patch of ground by marking it out with plaques, memorial stones or benches. If you do choose to scatter ashes in a 'garden of remembrance', the crematorium will keep a record of the exact site for the family. Indeed, the mourners can look forward to having their own ashes placed in that spot in the years to come.

> He didn't want to be buried, 'cos he didn't fancy that, and he didn't want to be remembered by those plants you see at the crematoriums, he didn't want to be remembered by no plant. So he wanted to be scattered, like what my Dad is. So they knew where my Dad had been scattered, although his ashes aren't there no more.
>
> (Christine)

Summary and conclusion

In this chapter I have focused on the strange balance between commerce and ritual. Within days of a death the survivors find themselves entering a new phase in the disposal of the deceased. Contact with the hospital, hospice or medical personnel stops. In its place a new relationship is gratefully forged with the funeral director. The surviving next of kin now find themselves involved in organizing the funeral as the focus turns towards the day of the service. The Reverend Ralph Peters' description of the funeral director as a master of ceremonies is a good one as they play a major role in our social organization of death.

As they endure the long wait between the day of the death and the day of the service the relatives find themselves making important financial decisions regarding coffins, mortuary clothes, flowers, stationery, food and drink for the wake, the hire of cars and the employment of funeral directors and members of the clergy. Most grieving families also make the emotional trip to the parlour to view the embalmed and encoffined corpse. During this staged and dramatic meeting, the funeral director remains firmly in charge, with the survivors finding themselves adopting the status of guest or visitor in a meeting with a member of their own family.

The day of the funeral is often met with some relief as the wait is over. Once again, it is the funeral director who ushers the family into the purring limousines to carry them to the local crematorium or cemetery. Participants derive different degrees of religious meaning from commital services and it is dangerous to generalize. In the course of my research I came across a wide spectrum of belief ranging from transcendental descriptions of rebirth at death to sad accounts of an empty and meaningless event. All services are short. Scarcely half-an-hour later the guests find themselves waiting for a lift to the deceased's home for the wake.

This is not the end of the story. Some months after the death many families choose to hold a memorial service. Most people also purchase memorials. Indeed, this represents something of a flourishing custom. There is a huge range of memorial artefacts on sale and you can spend a great deal of money on remembering the dead. Generally hidden behind the high walls of the cemetery or crematorium, it is easy to underestimate the important role that memorialization plays in our society.

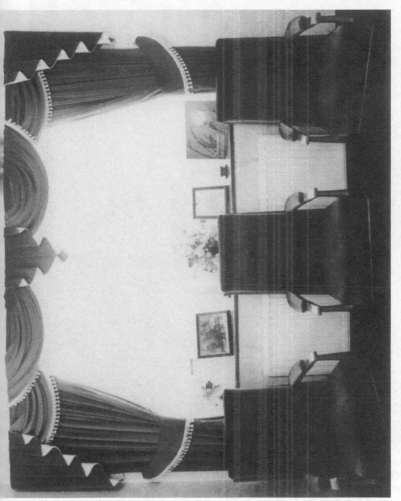

1. *Funeral parlour interviewing room* During the interview with the funeral director, grieving relatives make important decisions about the funeral, such as what the deceased will be wearing, the type of coffin they will use and whether they will be buried or cremated.

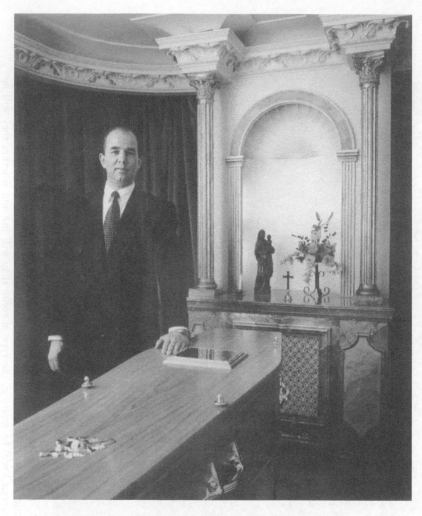

2. *Portrait of a funeral director*   Arguably, the most important person in the arrangement of contemporary funerals. Jeremy West, pictured here, is grandson of the founder of West and Co, an East End undertaking firm that currently arranges 2,400 funerals a year.

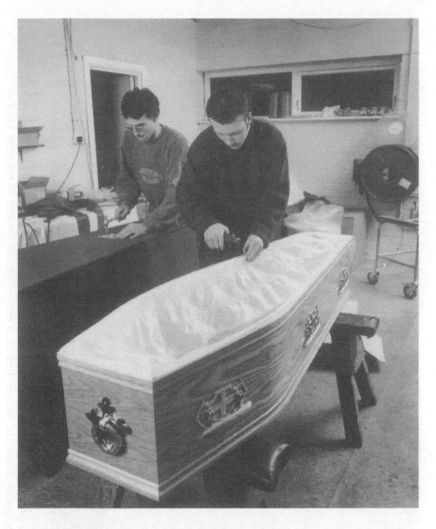

3. The coffin workshop Linings and fittings are being stapled and hammered in place. First lined with bitumen and polythene, the coffins are then embellished with satin and lace. Work proceeded to the beat of the radio. The notice board in this parlour was covered with letters of thanks from relatives.

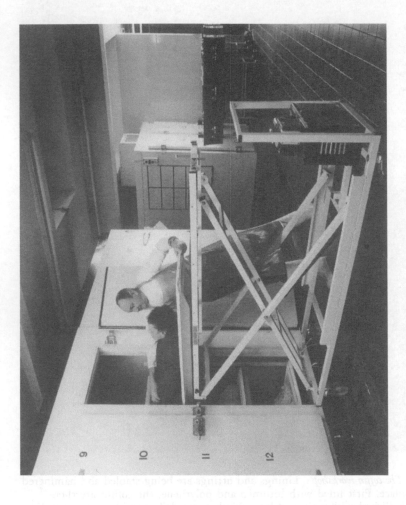

4. *Storage facilities in an embalming room* Having picked up the body from the hospital morgue or home, the funeral director is responsible for the care of the body prior to disposal. Nowadays most parlours keep the bodies in refrigerators.

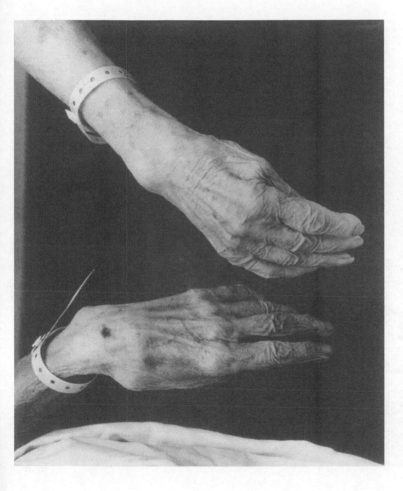

5. *Portrait of hands taken in an embalming room* This pair of beautiful old hands demonstrates the quite sriking contrast between embalmed and non-embalmed bodies. The woman on the right has been embalmed and you can see that the skin tone and texture is different to that of the hand on the left. After embalming, both of these corpses received a manicure.

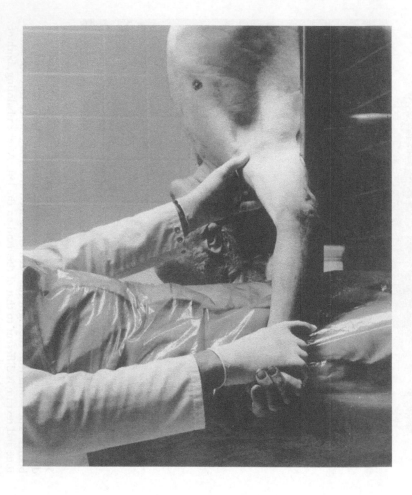

6. *An embalmer preparing a corpse* Here the embalmer is gently 'breaking up' the rigor mortis in a corpse, prior to embalming.

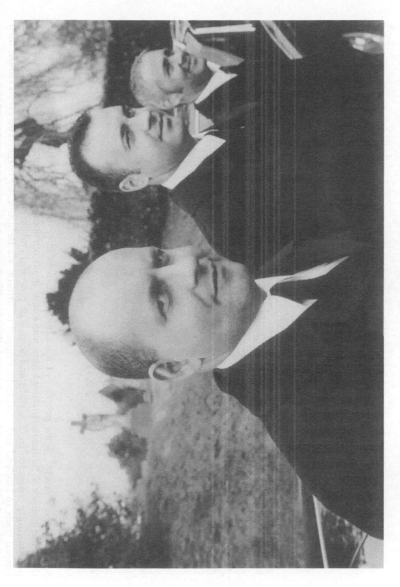

7. *Portrait of employees of an undertaking firm* Many men and women find their jobs in the 'death industry' enormously rewarding. I was often impressed by the sense of pride in the work. The serious and potentially depressing nature of the work is offset by a tradition of humour and camaraderie.

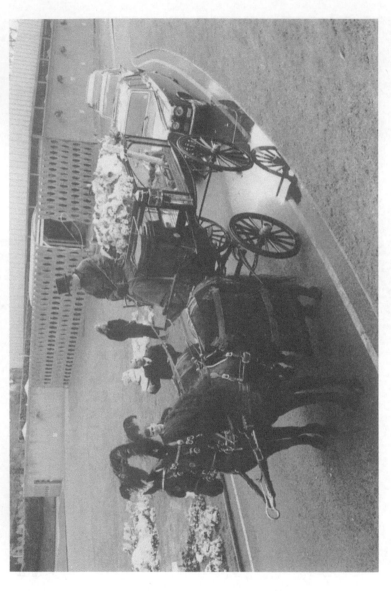

8. *Horse-drawn hearse* Some people opt for a horse-drawn hearse, the hire of which costs a little under a thousand pounds. The hearse pictured here was found in an outhouse in Epping in 1982 and was painstakingly renovated by T. Cribbs and Sons. The powerful and intensely black horses were bred for the funeral trade in Holland and used to be shipped to Britain, via Belgium, by barge. The breed almost died out during the second world war, although 'Belgian Blacks' are now enjoying a renaissance.

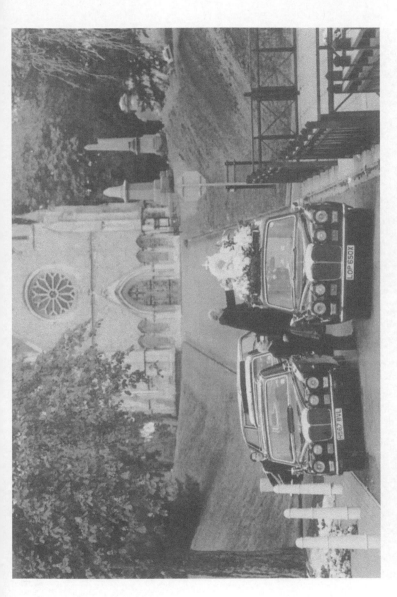

9. *Flower-covered hearse at a crematorium* Having driven to the crematorium or cemetery, the funeral director ushers the next of kin into the chapel. The undertakers then take the floral tributes and lay them on the 'floral display area', marked by personalised plaques. After the short service, which lasts for about half an hour, the relatives are directed to these arrangements to give them an opportunity to admire the flowers and read the accompanying cards.

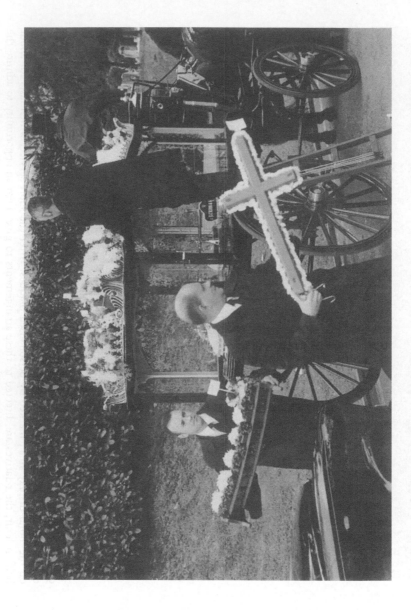

10. *Removing flowers from a horse-drawn hearse* Once again, floral tributes are being removed for display on the crematorium's floral tribute site. Flowers remain here until they begin to wilt.

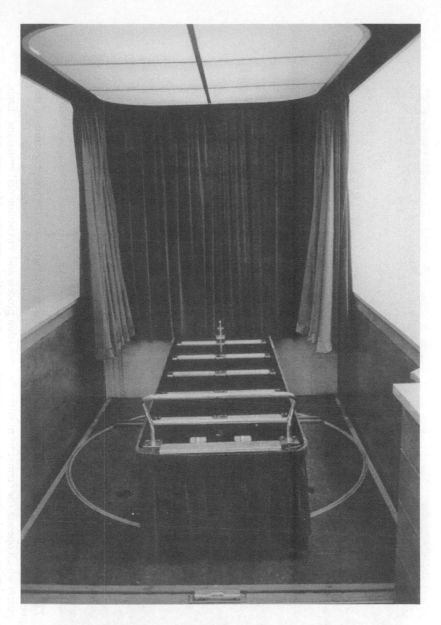

11. *The catafalque, temporary resting place of the coffin in the crematorium chapel* Once the relatives are seated, the funeral directors slowly carry in the coffin and place it upon the catafalque. In this modern crematorium, the automated curtain surrounds the coffin at the close of the ceremony. Later, once the relatives have left, the coffin is lowered to the ground floor for cremation, using the catafalque lift.

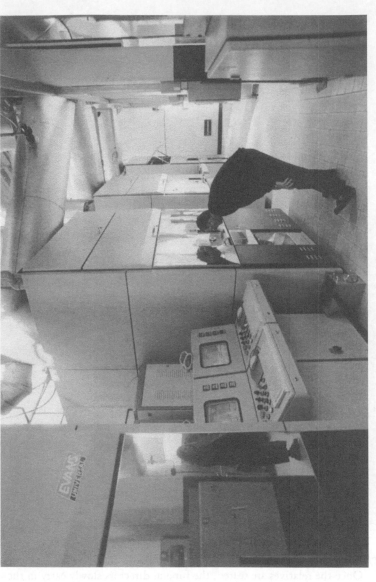

12. *The computer-operated cremators* The steel and ceramic contrast strongly with the softer textures of the chapels and gardens. These state of the art cremators cremate 4,000 to 4,500 'deceased' a year. The computers which operate the cremators monitor the cremation process and 'environmental emissions'. Each cremator has a peephole through which the 'operative' can monitor the cremation. After sixty minutes the computer will allow the operative to adjust the process if necessary.

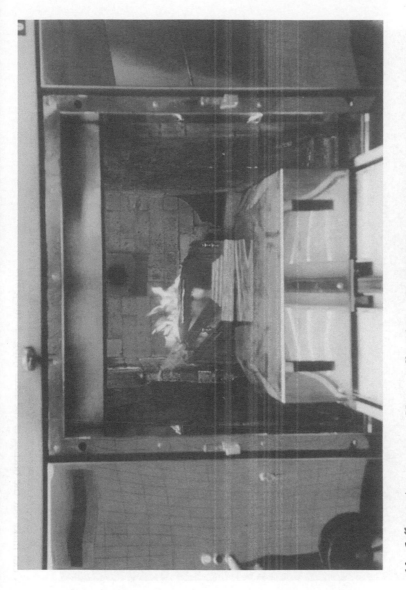

13. *Coffin entering a cremator* Here a coffin is being automatically pushed into a cremator. In the intense heat the coffin ignites immediately. The plastic handles soon melt away while the wood coffin contributes to the combustion of the corpse. After eighty minutes all that is left are the calcified remains.

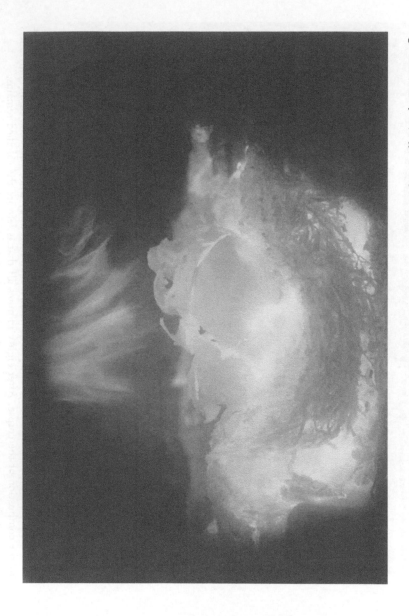

14. Photograph taken through cremator After half an hour or so, the wood of the coffin has burnt away. One can make out the outline of the skull lying on the pillow.

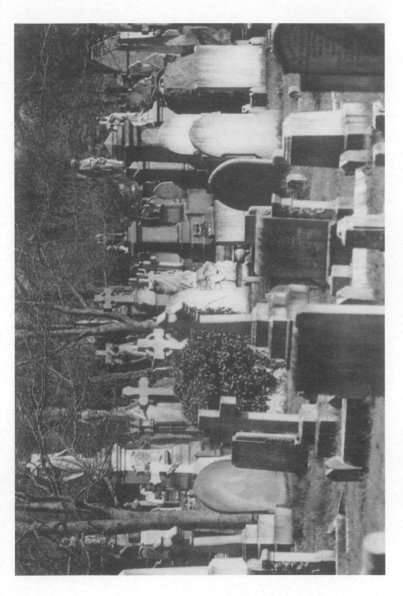

15. *Cemetery headstones*   While few of us can afford to purchase headstones such as the ones illustrated here, memorialisation continues to be an important part of our funeral rites. Reflecting the increasing appreciation of the importance of Britain's cemeteries, plans are afoot to conserve these headstones.

5 The body

An analysis of 'the body' represents something of a challenge to social psychologists, used to the study of psychological phenomena. In his exploration of the ill body Radley (1994) notes that being healthy or ill is not just an abstraction, but a physical reality. In this chapter I look at the dead body. I focus on the symbolic power of the threatening and unfamiliar corpse and ask whether our motivation for all that investigating, certifying and preserving, so often followed by the body's dramatic destruction by heat, is truly rational. I draw attention to the fact that contemporary death practices are processual; during the quite extended period of our death rites both the corpse and the grieving next of kin undergo certain transformations.

The ritual process

From the earliest days of anthropology, the analysis of mortuary rituals has dominated discussions of culture and society. Not only are most mortuary rituals flamboyant and striking in character, but they also tend to involve every member of a group and cause a suspension of normal day-to-day life. In non-industrial cultures, suffering from a high mortality rate, they also occur with great regularity.

In the West, technological innovation and rapid social change cause many people to feel nostalgic for the past. Indeed, many early anthropological observers became obsessed by a romantic vision in which 'primitive' peoples of the world were imagined to be living in some state of idealized natural bliss (Hockey 1996). Thus, 'science' and 'nature' were delicately counter-balanced. In many anthropological texts we can observe an implicit assumption that 'primitive man' was better off, spiritual and at one with his mortality. In short, the flamboyant and exotic funerals described were presumed to be functioning well. Here were 'life strategies' (Bauman 1992a) that worked.

In 1897 Durkheim (1952) set out to show that suicide, the apparently personal decision to take one's own life, was not an individual but a social act, demonstrated by the fact that different societies have different suicide rates. This was the inspiration for Hertz's 1905–6 (Hertz 1960) study of mortuary rituals of the Malayo–Polynesian people in which he attempted to show that death practices could be viewed as 'social facts'. Focusing on the collective representations of death, Hertz set out to demonstrate that grief, like suicide, was a social, rather than an individual, phenomenon. In his conception of things, death was envisioned as a threat to the fabric of society, something that presented a series of practical, social and metaphysical 'problems' to the survivors which could be solved through their participation in ritual. Such rituals served to separate the deceased from the world of the living before safely placing them in the world of the dead. During this period the deceased's soul was perceived to be dangerous and the mourners were seen to be at risk. These phases of disaggregation and reinstallation, expressed in this particular social group by temporary disposal and secondary burial respectively, represented a triumph of society over death. Hertz noted the similarity between such social transformations at death and those that take place at puberty and marriage, in which the participants undergo a change in their social identity (Bloch and Parry 1982).

A couple of years later Van Gennup, also a pupil of Durkheim, published his influential book *The Rites of Passage*. Van Gennup's (1960) study focused on those rituals that marked the life stages of birth, initiation, marriage and death. He argued that certain participants are transformed during these rituals, which are characterized by the themes of separation, liminality and reintegration. For example, during a funeral the deceased is separated from the community at death, remains in a limbo state for a while before being 'reborn' as an ancestor, spirit or ghost. As recently as 1982 Danforth applied Van Gennup's tripartite structure to the funeral practices in rural Greece. His work is relevant to the death practices described in the chapters that follow.

Bloch and Parry note that the sociological tradition of anthropology was not the only way in which death has been studied. A second tradition has focused on the symbolism of sexuality and fertility in mortuary practices (Bachofen 1967; Frazer 1980). Indeed, symbolic interpretations such as those provided by Bachofen in 1859 and Frazer in 1890 predated the study of social morphology but had not been fashionable. Bloch and Parry (1982) make use of both traditions in their fine discussion of beliefs of regeneration at death.

Like Frazer and Bachofen we are primarily interested in the way in which the symbolism of sexuality and fertility is used in the mortuary rituals; but with Hertz we share a concern with the social implications of mortuary practices, though not his view of society as an entity acting for itself. If we can speak of a reassertion of the social order at the time of death, this social order is a *product* of rituals of the kind we consider rather than their cause. In other words it is not so much a question of Hertz's reified 'society' responding to the 'sacrilege' of death, as of the mortuary rituals themselves being an occasion for *creating* that 'society' as an apparently external force.

(Bloch and Parry 1982: 6)

Using Leach's (1961) thesis concerning time being both repetitive and irreversible Bloch and Parry (1982) discuss how societies 'make believe' that death is an example of repetitive time. Death leads to life just as night leads to day. Societies create time using, for example, rituals and festivals to carve up the naturally continuous world into discontinuous and repetitive parts. Even an event as unpredictable as death can be used to articulate this play between repetitive and irreversible time. For example, Harris (1982) describes how in Latin America, the Laymi's all saints festival, which marks the beginning of the agricultural year, is a time when the deaths that have occurred throughout the year are ritually remembered. Thus the random distribution of death days are gathered into one significant celebration of the dead which, in turn, is an occasion to celebrate the fertility of the crops to come. Developing the theme of our efforts to control the arbitrariness of death, Bloch and Parry (1982) also draw attention to the relatively common practice of distinguishing between the physical death and the social recognition of the event. They note how certain deaths for the Lugbara peoples, for example, are defined as happening at the point when the dying person has spoken their last words to the heir. From that moment on the dying person is treated as if dead, suffering a social death.

In this chapter I shall apply these anthropological theories of transformations at death to contemporary funerals. There is a common assumption that contemporary funerals do not 'work'; these Western dysfunctional rituals are presumed to give rise to dysfunctional grief reactions. For many years the study of immortality in a Western context has been unfashionable. Discovering that people still believed in the afterlife does not seem to fit into the rationalist description of the world. Instead, Western funerals are often characterized as empty, their form shaped more by the forces of commerce and bureaucracy than by the need to ritually respond to the threat of death.

There are signs of change, however (see Bauman 1992a). Davies (1997) has looked at the similarities between contemporary cremation and the double burials first described by Hertz back in 1905. He traces the manner in which the identity of the corpse is not so much extinguished by cremation but transformed. In the first ritual the dead are removed from daily social life. In the second rite, the grieving relatives place the dead in the supernatural world of the ancestors. There is evidence to support the thesis that contemporary funerals do operate as rituals. The 'afterlife' does exist, although it may not necessarily conform to traditional conceptions of the other world. Thus along with the more traditional conceptions of heaven, we come across somewhat idiosyncratic versions of the world of the dead, peopled by ancestors. I would argue that such a conception is essential if we are going to understand the important role the dead play in our lives and I will discuss this at greater length in Chapter 7. How else are we going to explain the role played by the ubiquitous book of remembrance?

The corpse as a 'symbol system'

In almost every culture the ritual manipulation of the corpse provides a channel through which the survivors can articulate their systems of belief about society, life and death. Douglas (1966) noted how the living body can be used as a metaphor for society.

> The body is a model which can stand for any bounded system. Its boundaries can represent any boundaries which are threatened or precarious. The body is a complex structure. The functions of its different parts and their relation afford a source of symbols for other complex structures.
>
> (Douglas 1966: 115)

The body is both signifier and signified and Douglas notes a correlation between the ways in which people view their bodies and their society. For example, in a culture concerned with land and the dangers of invasion, maintaining the boundaries, or margins, of the group becomes an important issue. Invasion, the piercing of the boundary, is to be avoided at all costs. An obsession with territory and the maintenance of intact boundaries may be metaphorically expressed through a concern over the body's own boundaries, of skin and orifices. There may also be various customs pertaining to which kinds of food and drink can be imbibed. Alternatively, the release of and distribution of the body's products (particularly blood, semen, urine and faeces) may be surrounded by various prohibitions or social rules. Meanwhile, the unthinkable, invasion, may be ritually played-out and expressed through body-piercing. If the live body serves as such a rich symbol system, it makes sense that both the dying body and the corpse can also be utilized to express a group's concerns. Just as the live body can be used as a metaphor for the state of society, the corpse can also be brought into a metaphorical discourse.

The body can be used to express any aspect of the society. So the body can be used as a 'cognitive map through which we can discover the order of things in the external world' (Prior 1989: 17). In an industrial context, the body can become a metaphor for the Church, the state or, for that matter, medical science. Indeed, it is possible to chart the changes in the ways in which we conceive of the human form. During the nineteenth century the body was increasingly viewed as an object which could be investigated and observed as the fledgling medical sciences pinned pathology inside the human form. At the time when some were exploring the globe, medicine men came to see the body as a kind of atlas; knowledge of the body was taught as geography (Armstrong 1983). As Prior notes:

> Man the machine entered on stage and subsequently, this isolated, detached and mortal machine was viewed as a thing to be treated, reconstructed, repaired, improved and acted on.
>
> (Prior 1989: 9)

Armstrong (1983) traces the changes in medical writings reflecting reformulations of the nature and identity of the human body. Armstrong argues that it is possible to identify the shift from a nineteenth-century view of a discrete passive objective body to the twentieth-century relative and subjective body. During the course of this century there has been a new political anatomy at work that has turned the disembodied gaze from the body to the spaces between people. He argues we have constructed a 'web of investigation, observation and recording around individual bodies, their relationships and their subjectivity, in the name of health' (1983: 112).

> The new body is not a disciplined object constituted by a medical gaze which traverses it, but a body fabricated by a gaze which surrounds it; the new body is one held in constant juxtaposition to

other bodies, a body constituted by its social relationships and relative mental functioning, a body, of necessity, of a subject rather than an object.

(Armstrong 1983: 104)

Thus he argues that we can no longer view the doctor–patient relationship in nineteenth-century terms, as Foucault did (1973, 1979), as a clinical examination of a passive object. In the last few decades there have been many developments and now the doctor–patient relationship has been reinvented in terms of meaning, personality and compliance. The new patient, Armstrong argues, has been created out of these discourses. Exit man the machine, enter man the meaning-maker. This obsession with observing the spaces between bodies is reflected in the theory and methods of the social sciences; the exposure of 'truth' has become the new focus for research.

As Prior (1989) notes, the human form can be used in other ways, as a repository of human qualities, such as intelligence, or criminality or as a means of expression, typified by the study of non-verbal communication. Prior argues that it may be more useful to understand that what the body is 'depends on the very discourses that surround it' (1989: 18) (see also Foucault 1970, 1972).

In his discussion of the social organization of death in Belfast, Prior draws our attention to the central role played by the corpse. Thus the body 'also serves as a point on which private individuals can articulate their emotions, thoughts, practices and beliefs about death' (1989: 20). He makes the point that 'as far as the bereaved are concerned, the body is first and foremost a site of personhood: a point at which persona, social existence and the idiomatic soul interconnect' (1989: 20). My research findings support this point.

The signs of death are normally discovered 'on' or 'in' the body, the causes of death are invariably located deep inside the body, the registration of death is contingent on the production of a body, the bereaved weep over the body, the funeral director prepares the body, the clergy eulogise over an encoffined corpse. In fact, without a body the social processes that are contingent on death are severely and irreparably disrupted.

(Prior 1989: 13)

Order, disorder and dirt

In her examination of the ideas of pollution and of taboo Douglas (1966) explores how people order the universe through their selective perception and labelling of it. Those things that cannot be categorized according to our system of classification – those things that are inherently ambiguous – are often thought to be a source of pollution. They are dirt. Polluting objects, thoughts, people or animals can be responded to either negatively (ignored, not perceived, perceived and condemned) or positively (confronted). The latter response leads to a revision of our scheme of classification. Disorder, however, is not always either condemned or ignored. Indeed, participation in rituals represents a tacit recognition of the 'potency of disorder' (Douglas 1966: 94). Rituals, by confronting ambiguity, harness the power of this disorder and express the danger of ambiguity. An appreciation of the highly ambiguous nature of the corpse is the key to understanding why the body is a powerful symbolic object in human society. For here lies an object, of all objects, that is emotionally hard to categorize.

Douglas is at pains to demolish the myth that 'primitive' cultures and our own are completely different.

> If uncleanliness is matter out of place, we must approach it through order. Uncleanness or dirt is that which must not be included if a pattern is to be maintained. To recognise this is the first step towards insight into pollution . . . It involves no special distinctions between primitives and moderns: we are all subject to the same rules. But in the primitive culture the rule of patterning works with greater force and more total comprehensiveness. With the moderns it applies to disjointed, separate areas of existence.
>
> (Douglas 1966: 40)

She uses the example of 'shoes out of place'. Shoes are not dirty in themselves, she notes, but putting them on the dining-room table is a 'dirty' act.

> If we can abstract pathogenicity and hygiene from our notion of dirt, we are left with the old definition of dirt as matter out of place . . . Dirt is the by-product of a systematic ordering and classification of matter, in so far as ordering involves rejecting inappropriate elements.
>
> (Douglas 1966: 35)

Before decomposition sets in, a corpse can look not much different from a sleeping person. Yet closer inspection can throw an observer into confusion for, in contrast to a reposeful live body, the cold grey corpse is unmoving and unreactive. This object is ambiguous: clearly human in appearance, yet also clearly not human. We can begin to understand how the corpse contains a particularly strong power to pollute. Meanwhile, once the body starts to decompose it further challenges our senses of sight, smell and touch; it is easy to see why this somewhat gross physicality can be threatening to the survivors. The body's remorseless decay can be seen as a symbolic threat to the inner cohesion of a group. Thus many of the rituals of death and much of the symbolism about the dead are concerned with the corpse's transformation from the 'danger within' into an 'outside' object. In this process the group has an opportunity of restating its values, hierarchies and systems of belief. All in all, the corpse makes a great ritual object as it has the extraordinary power to surprise, shock or horrify.

As Douglas (1966) predicts, it is not easy to find a single comprehensive pattern of taboos and rules in a contemporary industrial society. Instead, we catch glimpses of pollution fears, concentrated in certain areas of ambiguity. So, in line with Douglas, I suggest that our ideas of pollution, far from being a just expression of deep-seated psychological fears or a response to the scientific facts of hygiene and pathogenicity, also express our social representations of the world. In fact, such an approach helps to explain apparent contradictions in our taboos about death that may otherwise be hard to understand. For example, I found that certain professionals, such as the mortuary attendant, pathologist and embalmer, who all manhandle the body, appear to become polluted by their contact while others who also have contact with the dead, such as the nurse and the doctor, do not. The pollution of the former group does not stem from their physical contact with the body itself, but from their perceived social role regarding the body. I will talk about the contagion of the professionals at greater length at the end of this chapter.

Women, sex and the decomposition of the flesh

Pertinent to any discussion of the symbolic power of the corpse is Bloch's (1982) analysis of the links between women, sex and the decomposition of the corpse. In an analysis of the way in which certain cultures view life as a 'limited resource', whereby each death makes way for another life, Bloch and Parry (1982) note that the regeneration of life can be viewed as a cause of death. For example, the Daribi believe that ejaculations deplete the life-force of men. Thus, death and reproduction are linked in the mind's eye and funerals are 'thoroughly permeated by the symbolism of rebirth' (1982: 9). From this, they expand their exposition to an analysis of the links between death, female sexuality, human reproduction and natural fertility. I suggest that these ideas are relevant to an examination of contemporary Western culture, however weakly stressed.

> Female sexuality is often associated with death only to be *opposed* to the 'real' fount of human and natural creativity; and that sexuality may be seen as the source of death and human pro-creation, which stands in opposition to non-human fertility.
>
> (Bloch and Parry 1982: 18)

Bloch and Parry suggest that certain non-industrial groups use gender symbolism to state the hierarchical contrast between sex and fertility; thus 'sexuality is set in opposition to fertility as women are opposed to men' (1982: 19). They illustrate their point with the Lugbara peoples, whose 'good' death will be discussed in the next chapter. For the Lugbara, they argue, fertility is envisioned as coming from the home-stead and from men, while sex is linked to women and the wilderness. For example, women are supposed to give birth outside the home-stead, in the bush. After the birth the women hand over the newborn child to the men, in the village.

> The symbolism of the mortuary rites of the Bara and Lugbara identifies women with sexuality, and sexuality with death. Victory over death – its conversion into rebirth – is symbolically achieved by a victory over female sexuality and the world of women, who are made to bear the ultimate responsibility for the negative aspects of death. In line with this, the sexuality of women is often closely associated with the putrescence of the corpse . . .
>
> (Bloch and Parry 1982: 22)

Expanding their thesis, Bloch and Parry argue that in certain cultures the sexuality of women may be linked to decomposition. A repetitive theme in many mortuary rituals is that the decay of the flesh is viewed as a necessary step before the soul can be released from the corpse. Bloch and Parry point to Strathern's (1982) study of the Gimi, where women 'consume' symbolic portions of the flesh of men's corpses to avoid the stage of decomposition altogether, thereby releasing their man's spirit immediately to the land of the ancestral spirits. Again, Bloch and Parry suggest that this emphasis on decomposition serves to emphasize the antithesis: rebirth.

To reiterate: death is transformed into rebirth and this can be dramatically established through rituals that often use gender symbolism to state a victory of men, fertility and rebirth over women, sex and decomposition. In this instance, Bloch and Parry suggest that this symbolism is used to keep those in power in control.

> Society is made both emotionally and intellectually unassailable by means of that alchemy which transforms death into fertility. This fertility is represented as a gift made by those in authority which they bestow by their blessings.
>
> (Bloch and Parry 1982: 41)

Bloch and Parry (1982) are examining non-Western cultures, yet it is possible that the same themes continue to exist in our own culture. Some examples I have given may appear bizarre or exotic, yet the underlying representations of sex, women and death may not be as foreign as they appear at first glance; the links between sex and death in the West have been noted before (Gorer 1955). In a fascinating analysis of representations of the dead female form in Western art, Bronfen (1992) brings the symbolic role of women in death closer to home. Using Gabriel Von Max's 1869 kitsch painting, *Der Anatom*, she explores some of the messages that are sent by this extraordinary image of the naked female corpse of a beautiful young woman who is under the steady gaze of an anatomist, poised to start his work. As Bronfen wryly notes, this woman is the perfect object, being dead. Her beauty is made more rare by the observer's knowledge that she will soon be cut by the anatomist's knife. Here we see all the ingredients of patriarchy offering society a form of immortality via scientific knowledge. The middle-aged anatomist has triumphed over the eroticized female form that lies before him. Of course, we undertake a dangerous confrontation with death by looking at this picture. But to some extent this danger is neutralized by the fact that, like the anatomist, what we gaze on is the other. Bronfen argues that in Western culture the superlative site of otherness is the feminine body. We are therefore offered the opportunity of distancing death one step further. Thus representations of beautiful dead women in art, such as Millais' *Ophelia* (1851–2), can be viewed not only as a symptom of a repression that fails (Bronfen 1992), but also as a triumph of men over women.

In the following section, I return to the acts of post-mortem, embalming, viewing, burial and cremation. I focus on how our in-articulate ideas of purity and dirt lie beneath the surface of our social organization of death. I illustrate the ways in which fears of pollution from the decomposing corpse and the strength of taboos around death and decay are harnessed to create and maintain male power and authority. In the course of this discussion I also reveal the gradual changes that come over the two travellers, the dead and those that survive them, in this ritual process.

The dead in the world of the living

In Chapter 3 I drew attention to the fact that even the timing of the actual moment of death has become an area of uncertainty and the subject of fierce debate (Glover 1990). With the advent of sophisticated medical tools and techniques, such as the use of life-support systems, the identification of the start of the post-mortem period is not always easy. We could argue that even 'the moment of death' is a cultural construction. As Brown (1987) points out, our definition of 'deadness' is changing as our understanding of physiology advances. In the quotation below, the Reverend Ralph Peters talks about his time as a hospital chaplain. He is describing the tragic death of three young men.

> I saw them up in ITU and . . . they were brain stem dead. And what got me particularly, was to see these three young men . . . without a scratch, mark, blemish, bruise on their bodies. . . . Physically they were whole and fit and perfect specimens, you could say . . . And yet, because of the brain-stem death there was nothing functioning from here [neck] upwards . . . And that really got to me, a) because they were so young, and so it was a premature death but b) because there was no physical symptom, if you like, there was no injury, there were no cancerous cells, there was merely a technical injury . . . And, in a sense, I suppose, if a person is dying or dead they ought to show it in their features in some way. Either look very grey or look at peace, if they had been through a lot of illness, or be very . . . aged and wrinkled . . . But if there is nothing physically there to indicate that this person is dying or dead, somehow you can't marry the knowledge of their death with the physical presence in front of you.
>
> (The Reverend Ralph Peters)

In the first few hours after a death we can observe a dramatic change in the way that people who have care of the body treat it. But their response to the newly dead is by no means uniform. There are a whole range of responses to the polluting potential of the dead body and much depends on the physical condition of the corpse. A brain-stem dead person kept alive on a life-support machine, while rationally being accepted by staff and kin alike as 'dead', very often appears not to be emotionally accepted as physically dead (and thereby polluting). These corpses are generally too 'whole' to fall into the dangerous category. The body of a dead person who is being ventilated presents the observers with a strange and confusing image (Robbins 1996). Such bodies are treated more like patients than corpses. These warm, pink and breathing bodies are not so polluting. Indeed, the organs of this 'non-dead' corpse can be put into the living bodies of others through transplant surgery.

The philosophical questions raised by organ donation are not simple to answer. In a fascinating analysis of the sociological questions raised, Robbins (1996) notes the contrast in public feeling between 'living donations' (blood, sperm, milk, plasma) and the extraction of products from the dead. Demand for organs for transplantation exceeds supply and waiting lists are notoriously long. Robbins (1996) notes that various monetary and non-monetary rewards have been paid to donor families for organs in some countries. Back in 1996 Richardson drew attention to similarities between the quest for organs in the twentieth century and the search for corpses for dissection in the eighteenth century. With haunting prescience she noted that the conditions for the emergence of an international black market in organs appeared to be in place. In Britain, keeping a fresh supply coming from intensive care units seems to be dependent on periodic publicity drives which either emphasize our moral duty or evoke our sympathy by describing the plight of the chronically ill awaiting new organs. These efforts to suppress our pollution taboos regarding the dead's organs are a salient aspect of modern transplant surgery.

When advanced technology is not involved, the business of defining death is usually easier. In such instances the change from person to corpse is obvious to all. Doctors, nurses and the bereaved next of kin described the state of a newly dead body as being familiar. The body could be mistaken for a person asleep. However, within hours, signs of decomposition become apparent. I suggest that the threat of the impending decomposition of the corpse gives rise to this feeling that this recently stilled body is 'matter out of place'. The body is dangerous and powerful. In an industrial, urban context, having become unused to the life cycle in the raw, it makes sense that we may attempt to control death – to hide, stem and then destroy altogether any signs of decomposition.

There is almost this defence mechanism, which turns round and says, 'Well, I am picking up an arm, or a leg, or a piece of meat here' . . . but that is not a dead body any more, because you can look into the butcher's window and see more gruesome sights, to be honest with you.

(Inspector Brown)

I have become much more hardened over a post-mortem now. I am now coping with the fact that it is just a piece of meat.

(Inspector Baker)

Seen in these terms, it is easy to see how a disfigured body may set up very complex reactions. Like the decomposing corpse it is confusing and threatening, human and yet not human. If the body has suffered very severe damage, it may be hard to recognize it as human at all. If the body is mutilated then it is unlikely that relatives will get access to the corpse, or what remains of it (see page 130).

The modern Western response to mortality is to set in motion a series of investigative procedures in order to discover why a death occurred (Prior 1989: 13). We can observe a rush to categorize. Only certain professionals are qualified to undertake this labelling. In the quotation below, a police inspector is acknowledging the primacy of the medical profession.

We can't assume death, even if you have got a head over there and a body over there, it is not dead until somebody comes along and says 'He is dead'.

(Inspector Brown)

Prior (1989) notes how this quest, which is directed towards the diseased or damaged organ seen as responsible for death, can lead to difficulties because, 'for many individuals, several pathological conditions will be present at the moment of death. Indeed, it may sometimes be the case that it is the simultaneous occurrence of diseases which causes death rather than any single affliction' (Prior 1989: 91). The death certificate is not viewed by clinicians as a potential source of clinical data but as a medico-legal document. In many ways, the certification of the dead is just 'paper work'.

All deaths have causes, each death has a cause, each particular death has its particular causes. Corpses are cut open, explored, scanned, tested until *the cause* is found; a blood clot, kidney failure, haemorrhage, heart arrest, lung collapse. We do not hear of people dying of mortality. They die only of individual *causes*, they die because *there was an individual cause*.

(Bauman 1992b: 138)

Certainly this was supported by my research, where one doctor admitted that her form-filling represented a mere estimate of the cause of death. If particularly busy, she sometimes did not even examine the corpse. While this is understood among medical practitioners, the bereaved public take the cause of death written on the form seriously. What we have here is a form of social behaviour that is not so much about identifying a 'real' cause of death, but which serves the purpose of creating a semblance of order at the time of death. Perhaps our efforts to identify the cause, to put a handle on death, are not so very different from those of tribal people who attribute deaths to witchcraft or evil spirits?

Viewing the embalmed

Embalming . . . makes the deceased look better and removes infection. And, therefore, danger.

(Funeral Director, Hart's Funeral Parlour)

The manipulation of the corpse to enhance its appearance has a great deal in common with our efforts to beautify the living body (Foltyn 1996). Gender plays an important role here. In her analysis of beautiful female dead during the eighteenth century Bronfen (1992) argues that the relatively new practice of embalming offered the survivors an opportunity to enjoy a continuing ownership of the corpse as 'other'. They could gaze on this perfect object for as long as they pleased. In these instances the beautiful embalmed body resembled art in so far as 'it has no relation to the world in which it appears except that of an image, of a shadow' (1992: 104). For, hauntingly, the corpse's 'point of references is ultimately nothing' (1992: 104). This insight goes some way in helping to explain the extreme discomfort that can be felt in the presence of the embalmed dead.

But. Whoever I have seen [embalmed] I don't like. They are not that person. You know. I know they . . . they embalm and all that, but they are not the same person, the way they do them up.

(Janet)

C. Davies (1996) has noted that the cult of hygiene, youth and beauty is more strongly articulated in the United States than it is here. Plastic surgery, although gaining in popularity in the UK, is still more widespread in America. Further, C. Davies (1996) notes the American obsession for personal cleanliness, expressed by high sales of deodorants. She suggests that, in death, there is a similar concern for presenting an odourless self. Drawing on an analysis of 'otherness' engendered by waves of immigration in the late nineteenth and early twentieth century in which play was made between being a 'clean' American citizen and a 'dirty' migrant, she argues that the hygienic all-American citizen would quite naturally choose sanitizing embalming as part of their post-mortem practices. While there are certain transatlantic differences in the approach to embalming which reflect trends among the living, it appears that the same basic processes are at work. The same themes of beauty, restoration, hygiene and denial were apparent in my analysis of British embalming practices although I suggest that they are probably less strongly articulated.

> Embalming restores a much more pleasant appearance . . . as far as the family are concerned, it gives people a more healthy appearance. One of being at rest, rather than one of being – dead.
> (Funeral Director, Haynes' Funeral Homes)

Yet another motive behind the manipulation of the dead is that of altering the form of death. This was particularly apparent when the cause of death resulted from disfiguring accidents. Embalmers were often engaged in quiet deceits in their efforts to give the impression to the deceased's relatives that the manner of death was less violent than was the case. We often talk about the ideal 'good death' of passing away in our sleep. Presenting the bereaved family and friends with an image of that 'sleeping corpse' – irrespective of the way the person actually met their end – is a way of pretending that that person died in a calm and peaceful way. In the next chapter I will discuss more fully the close link between the idea of the good death and the cause of death and I will claim that our efforts to embalm are an overt expression of this link. Thus a disfiguring death after a traffic accident – a bad death – will cause the embalmer to try to improve the state of the corpse as they strive to remove all signs of the deceased's violent end.

> I once spent eight hours embalming a person. I had to suture an arm back on – the relatives didn't know that they had lost an arm.
> (Funeral Director, Dent's Funeral Parlour)

Refrigeration in itself only slows down decomposition, and doesn't actually stop decomposition. Whereas embalming does. If a body is embalmed fully, it can literally last a lifetime.

(Funeral Director, Haynes' Funeral Homes)

Embalming is something of a quirky custom. While it is true that the preservation of a corpse may reduce the risks of infection and will certainly reduce the odour and other unpleasant side-effects of decomposition, it is also true that the same advantages can be achieved by the simpler process of rapid disposal. Hallam *et al.* (forthcoming) draw attention to the inherent contradictions involved in tampering with the decomposing corpse and note:

> By re-establishing the body's boundaries, workers come into direct contact with the most dangerous of the body's polluting products: blood, mucous and excreta. In bolstering up the boundaries of the flesh and presenting the deceased as undamaged and intact, the techniques adopted are themselves violent and transgressing of those very boundaries. The restoration of order therefore needs to be understood as something which operates most powerfully at the symbolic level.
>
> (Hallam *et al.* forthcoming)

A common theme in cultures across the world is the desire to manipulate the corpse to maintain some vestige of control over the chaos of death. Many cultures are content to leave the body – often viewed as a mere empty shell – as it stands. Other groups are keen to speed up this process of decay (Strathern 1982). Bloch (1982) has discussed the elaborate ways in which the Merina, in Madagascar, strive for the achievement of the skeletal – dry – state of the corpse. In our culture we want to prolong the corpse's fleshy – wet – state. In the process, it is not just the corpse that undergoes a transformation, but also the participants who experience a series of subtle alterations in their roles and statuses, not to mention the changes wrought to their social representations of life and death.

> If you think of the word, 'embalm', means balm, sweetness, gentleness. And that is what we aim at.
>
> (Mr Molesworth, Molesworth's Funeral Parlour)

So what are we saying when we fill a corpse's arteries with formaldehyde and sew the mouth closed? The act of embalming is not dissimilar to surgery or to a post-mortem. The embalmer works in a room that apes the appearance of a hospital theatre and they make use of 'medical' tools and substances. Thus, in keeping with the dominant ideologies and beliefs of our time, embalming fits nicely into the domain of medical-type interventions. In these terms tinkering with the body–object is no contradiction: it is simply yet another expression of the now familiar and comforting model of man the machine, fixable, as long as we have the skill. Embalming can be viewed as a strategy whereby we attempt to attain some kind of mastery over death. However, despite their efforts, this control can still be tenuous. One funeral director to whom I spoke talked of 'rogue corpses' that, strangely, decay in a noxious way, despite being embalmed.

Behind these actions lies another motive, unique to an industrial culture and connected to the professionalization of death. Embalming is a good way of charging more money. More bodies are embalmed than are viewed which seems to undermine some funeral directors' arguments that this is done solely for the benefit of the bereaved. Referring to the quotation below, I would imagine that the threat of an 'unpleasant' corpse would be enough to encourage even the most resistant client to agree to have their loved one embalmed.

> I can't promise that in the time between the death and the funeral that nothing unpleasant will happen. If they have been embalmed, I can say 'Yes, nothing unpleasant will happen.'
> (Funeral Director, Dent's Funeral Parlour)

The trip to the funeral director's viewing 'chapel' to see the embalmed corpse is a relatively new custom. In the past friends and family gathered around the dying person. After a death a second gathering took place just before the funeral, at the wake, in which the then encoffined body had pride of place. Normally the lid would be closed after the wake. In the last 100 years or so, as the funeral director took over control of the body, it became necessary for the bereaved to make a visit to the corpse who, previously, would have been at the family's own home. The brief trip to the funeral director's chapel appears to be a survival of an old social custom, altered to suit the constraints of the professionalization of death.

> When I went down to view him, my neighbour came with me. And I just froze. I just couldn't go in there. I just couldn't go in – and Peter [the funeral director] he was there and, well this is a bit cruel, but he just forced me, he just pushed me in there. It was a

bit cruel. He just said 'You'll regret it later if you don't do this' and he just pushed me. I had wanted to go, but when I got there I just couldn't.

(Christine)

I found that funeral directors often referred to 'lay' psychological models of grief to explain why it was important for the bereaved to view. While I was in the field several parlours were considering publishing customized grief handbooks for their customers. These booklets are based on somewhat simplistic stage–phase models of 'grief work'. Viewing the embalmed body was presumed to jog the grieving person out of the stage of 'numbness' into the next phase, that of, say, 'depression and despair'.

This is all very well for 'good deaths' but 'bad deaths' were construed as being bad for the grief reaction. Several funeral directors told me that viewing damaged corpses not only caused immediate trauma but also that this could lead to a bad (pathological) grief outcome. The funeral director's power in these instances should not be underestimated. Funeral directors try hard to stop the next of kin from viewing damaged bodies. One director boasted to me that he intervened in an instance where a woman wanted to say goodbye to her husband's body after his sudden death. The corpse was disfigured. The director had a 'chat' with the woman's doctor and the doctor 'successfully' dissuaded her from viewing the body. Their motivation for doing so finds its source in the assumption that the role of viewing is to reassure the relatives that the mode of death was a good one, and not to register the fact of death. For, if it were the latter, the state of the corpse would be immaterial – if you are dead you are dead. This seems to echo Prior's findings in Belfast. He noted that funeral directors feel that corpses that 'cannot be sculptured into restful and peaceful poses . . . are "bad remains"' (Prior 1989: 161). In similar vein, discussing viewings for identification purposes a coroner talked of allowing relatives unused to seeing the dead to do identifications only if the body were to 'lie there serenely asleep'.

Susan had been abroad when her husband had died. Although she had been able to visit the hospital mortuary this had not been a good experience. His body had not been prepared in any way; he was still half-dressed and his head was covered in blood. She was particularly distressed because she could not easily touch her husband's body which was displayed behind a glass partition.

He flung back the curtains, and Max was lying there with a glass partition half opened, so you could get access only to the top half of Max's body. With a sheet turned back, and he was still wearing his trousers and braces . . . I wanted to kiss him . . . and, you know, everything in you wants to put your arms right, right round him.

(Susan)

Robbed of any opportunity to say farewell to him at his moment of death, access to his body was of great importance to her. Going to the funeral parlour to spend some time with him and take stock of what had happened was, she felt, good for her.

I sat in their small chapel . . . simply furnished with the coffin . . . And I took some flowers from the garden . . . and I sat there for an hour, and that was a very good hour.

(Susan)

There are other reasons why people view their dead relatives. Earlier I was discussing the fearful trade of corpses for dissection (see p. 11). An age-old anxiety concerning the fate of the corpse and a slight distrust of the director's competence or scrupulousness appears to live on. Janet was particularly concerned to view her husband's body as he had died while they were on holiday in the countryside. She was worried that his body would have somehow become muddled up with someone else on the journey home.

The reason why I wanted to view was to make sure they had the right person. That was really my thoughts all along – you are the only person I have told this to! – I thought, well, you hear of so many mix-ups, you know, I wanted to make sure.

(Janet)

Funeral directors, having aspired to embalm the body into a sleep-like appearance, set the body for viewing in a posture that dates from the middle ages. Eyes and mouth are closed, the body is placed on its back, arms at its side. The body may be dressed in personal formal clothes, or may wear a coffin shroud. From the funeral director's point of view, viewing provides them with an opportunity to show off their handiwork. I could often detect suppressed pride in their work. They have proved their power over the ravages of death.

A triumph of society over death?

Leaney (1989) has observed that there seems to be an apparent contradiction between the act of embalming, to preserve, followed by the act of cremation, to destroy. But this is not seen as a contradiction within the industry.

> If we allowed the decomposition of the corpse preceding the clean cremation it would make the whole point of cremation a waste of time.
>
> (Funeral Director, Hart's Funeral Parlours)

We can see that the medical model has extended well into the post-mortem period. As I noted on p. 85, the backstage areas of some crematoria simulate a hospital ward or a mortuary. Again, cremation chimes well with our desire for human control over death by medical science.

Having made the dead look as if they died the good death, we state our control over death by destroying our handiwork altogether. Is it not possible that we are attempting to create the illusion that it is not death who is the player in this drama, but the embalmer and the crematorium attendant? The artificial destruction of the corpse is attractive precisely because it bypasses nature. To put it another way, cremation destroys the corpse before it gets to look too bad. Further support for this thesis is supplied by D. J. Davies (1996) who uncovered fascinating gender differences in the preference for cremation over burial. He found that twice as many of his female respondents expressed a dislike for burial. He suggests that women, whose self-identity has been forged with the appearance of their bodies, may be choosing cremation over burial to avoid the disturbing fantasy of the ugly and repulsive rotting female form. The quick cremation rite offers the opportunity of avoiding such identity-threatening imagery. The cremation of the body offers the promise of the instant removal of the decaying, polluting, flesh.

I asked deathworkers why they thought people choose cremation over burial. I still remember one funeral director leaning back in his chair thoughtfully before replying with the statement 'Cremation is cleaner and more advantageous.' I am still unsure about his precise meaning of 'advantageous', but the implied contrast this director made with the polluting power of dirty burial is quite clear. Another funeral director argued that the choice of cremation was connected to a commitment to the 'green movement', i.e. the saving of wasted (and presumably symbolically polluted) land. The logic does not necessarily follow as there are concerns that the combustion of certain glues and plastics used in coffins can create local pollution.

So, miraculously, the rotting corpse is transformed into dry ashes, safely contained in a pot. Yet from the bereaved families' point of view the act of cremation is unlikely to feel like any kind of victory of human control over death. Indeed, they can feel quite the reverse: that the cremation of the dead seems strangely cold.

> I don't know, it was so dismal. The idea of this casket, you know, being reduced to ashes . . . We went there directly after the funeral. But that didn't worry me a bit. The thing that did upset me was interring the ashes, some months later. I didn't like that one bit.
>
> (Beth)

As Beth succinctly put it, the cremation was 'just the technical bit'. Other women also expressed reserved feelings about the cremation rite. This is not surprising when we consider that they did not know very much about the business of cremation. The cremation of the body takes place backstage and most relatives are not even sure at what time the body would have been cremated.

Crematoria are extremely careful to maintain the integrity of each set of ashes. Contrary to popular myth, there is no promiscuous mixing of remains: apparently a gross and disturbing thought in this individualistic culture. After each cremation the ashes are carefully collected and labelled before being stored in neat rows, awaiting their request from the relatives. Ashes, or 'cremains' as they are known within the trade, have great symbolic power and my subjects usually had strong feelings about them. As I mentioned in the last chapter, crematoria are aware of such sentiments, providing a 'holding service'. They will guard the ashes, for a small fee, until their bereaved client feels able to decide how they would like to dispose of them.

The scattering, burial or storing of ashes can evoke strong emotional responses for the next of kin. While many eventually choose to let the staff at the crematorium scatter the ashes within their walls, others improvise, creating their own private and, at times, powerful rituals. People scatter the ashes in favourite holiday sites, on mountain tops, in rivers, at birth sites, etc. Earlier I was discussing Hertz's (1907, translated in 1960) analysis of double rituals in some societies in which efforts are made to distinguish between the first rite to remove the wet flesh, symbolically representing the removal of the deceased from the world of the living, to the second rite in which the dry bones or ashes are disposed of, in which the deceased enters a new phase as it enters the world of the dead. Davies (1997) has applied Hertz's theory to contemporary cremation and the widespread custom of scattering the ashes in some site of personal and private sentimental value. Davies draws our attention to the fact that the modern day secondary disposal of the ashes affords the survivors the opportunity not only of signalling the deceased's entry into the world of the ancestors, but also of being involved in what he calls a 'retrospective fulfilment of the identity of the lost partner' (D. J. Davies 1996: 27).

> Cremation has introduced this optional rite where the single mourner takes the cremated remains of partner, child or friend and locates them wherever desired. This marks a new ritual process in the modern Western world.
>
> (Davies 1997: 29)

Davies notes the huge variation across the country between the percentage of cremains that are taken out of the crematoria for scattering or interment elsewhere. Davies compares the rate of removal of 67 per cent in Bodmin to the modest 18 per cent in south London. It is possible that regional differences could partly be explained by ease of access to good dramatic countryside in which to conduct these rituals of reincorporation.

Burial, in contrast, appears to be viewed by the general public and deathwork professionals alike as natural. Decomposition in the soil – a messy process – takes time. It also does not need help from mankind. I found that even after decomposition has taken place the buried dead continue to have the power to pollute and to threaten. It appears they can even pollute each other. For example, one cemetery manager told me of a client who insisted that her husband's body was surrounded by 'virgin' soil: soil that came from outside the polluted cemetery. The strength of such feelings seemed to suggest that efforts to launch rapid recycle plots, in which the remains are removed a few years after burial, in overcrowded urban cemeteries would meet with some deep resistance from the general public. It is of note that in America the 'burial' of the dead actually involves putting caskets in metal or concrete vaults so that the casket has no contact with the earth (C. Davies 1996).

We can begin to unravel degrees of pollution, too. For example, I was told by staff from two cemeteries of times when relatives asked for the exhumation of the dead from 'common graves' because they had not realized that meant their loved one would share a grave with other people. One cemetery manager told me that people got more upset if the graves contained corpses from different ethnic groups, not just a case of 'matter out of place', but 'people out of place'. It appears that we are witnessing some kind of racist hierarchy of pollution fears. While certain people may find their own dead relative to be highly polluting, that corpse is less polluting than the dead body of a non-family member from the same ethnic group which, in turn, is less polluting than the dead body of a person from another ethnic group. Sadly, death may not always be such a great leveller.

The contamination of the survivors

This review of current death practices reveals quite complex fears of pollution. Given such feelings, it hardly comes as a surprise to find that those who have close contact with the dead – the deathwork professionals – can be contaminated by their proximity to the ambiguous corpse.

I distinctly remember when I met an embalmer on a working day. The impulse to wipe my hand having shaken hands with him was almost impossible to master. Professionals who physically handle the dead are the most obvious candidates for contamination. However, as I mentioned earlier, I was interested to note how this contamination does not seem to affect those who touch the very newly dead: namely the doctor and nurse. Although an explanation can be found in the non-acceptance of the body as dead, it is also a function of the way in which nurses and doctors are not acknowledged, within the medical and public realms, as deathworkers. The mortuary attendant, who also touches the fresh corpse, along with the pathologist, the embalmer and the cremator attendant are highly contaminated by their contact. Thus the binary opposition between life and death is extended to the professionals who deal with 'saving life' and those who 'deal in death'. Giving expression to this split, one patients' affairs officer did not like the waiting relatives to see visiting funeral directors and organized her appointments accordingly. This elaborate precaution was quite strange as the self-same next of kin would often combine their sub-sequent visit to the register office with a trip to the funeral parlour. As far as the patients' affairs officer was concerned, funeral directors did not belong in hospitals.

The contamination of those professionals who deal in death is given expression through their isolation and their exclusion from direct contact with the bereaved. They become 'untouchable'. Such is the way we organize death, that the 'untouchable' professionals rarely meet the bereaved client. This is achieved through the architectural design of buildings and through bureaucratic and administrative procedures. Again we return to the theme of the front and back of house as elaborated by Goffman (1961). Many of the 'untouchable's' activities – of post-mortem, embalming and cremating – take place 'backstage', where no kin can observe what happens, in sites that are themselves highly contaminated.

In many smaller firms, the funeral directors themselves embalm in the back of the parlours. They tend to keep quiet about their work-shops and their activities therein, alternating uncomfortably between the incompatible roles of 'untouchable' and a kind of funereal tourist guide for the bereaved. Although funeral directors who do not embalm and whose roles are, for all practical purposes, consistently 'front of house' may still experience the effects of contamination. Two funeral directors to whom I spoke expressed the problems they had, during social engagements, when members of the public became aware of their profession.

> I prefer, now, to say I am a company director if people ask me what I do, rather than say I am a funeral director. It depends where I am and who I am with. I used to have guitar lessons, and one day the teacher asked me what I did for a living. She wouldn't teach me afterwards.
>
> (Funeral Director, Dent's Funeral Parlour)

Fear of pollution is not only expressed in behaviour, it is also expressed in talk. Funeral directors remain past-masters in the art of euphemism. In the trade, among funeral directors, 'doing a proper job' involves avoiding unpleasant – polluting – words like 'dead' and 'deceased'. A director from Dent's Funeral Parlour argued that 'there is no need' to call the dead 'deceased' or refer to their 'body', as one can simply refer to their kinship tie with the client, i.e. 'your mother', 'your son'.

> I avoid the word 'deceased', so I say 'Can I have the person's name' – presuming they will understand who I mean.
>
> (Funeral Director, Haynes' Funeral Homes)

Half-way through my interview with Ann she looked me in the eye and informed me that I was sitting on her husband's chair. It is not just the deathwork professional who can become subject to fears of pollution. Such feelings about the dead person's possessions, body or remains can initiate terrible guilt. When people die at home their relatives may be challenged by ambivalent feelings. Eleanor was still not sleeping in the room where her husband had died when I interviewed her nine months later. The problem of the contagious nature of physical remains resurfaces when the bereaved are asked if they wish to take the ashes home. Both the professionals and the bereaved talked about the problems of having the ashes at home. Eleanor, apparently, could not stand the idea of polluting her home in this way so she asked her daughters to pick them up from the funeral directors for her. Fearing censorship and being loath to pay the rental fee, Kate never told her family that she had stored her husband's ashes in a cupboard. Unlike Eleanor, Kate did not seem to mind this close contact with her husband's remains but she was not immune to the imagined horror of others if they were to hear that her husband's 'cremains' sat tucked away with her shoes.

The bereaved friends and family are contaminated in a quite different way as they do not manhandle the body on a professional basis but caress it with familiarity and affection.

> [The nurse] told me to hold his hand, and I know he looked like he was sleeping . . . After about ten minutes I did do it.
>
> (Christine)

The bereaved's gentle strokes, embraces and kisses, however fleeting, can also leave them mildly 'tainted' in other people's eyes. The response of others to the bereaved's contamination is much the same as it is to the 'untouchable' professional. They are isolated. This can be expressed physically or emotionally. The widows talked about the way certain people avoided them since the deaths of their husbands. They put this down to a certain social embarrassment, which is probably true, but I also suggest that this could be an expression of a fear of contamination.

> There were two neighbours who behaved all right. [But] they were all scared. One of them came and sat here, he was petrified.
>
> (Ruth)

Another source of fear regarding those suffering from grief stems from the 'asocial' behaviour typical of someone experiencing such intense sorrow. People are simply not as predictable, or as polite, as they formerly were. For those unaffected by a death the bereaved can appear unreliable and over-emotional. This volatility is quite understandable, for besides the pure sorrow of loss, a bereaved person may find their very sense of self has been altered by the death. One registrar I interviewed passionately believed that the bereaved should wait to register the death of their loved one in separate waiting rooms. This was not just a question of giving sorrowing individuals privacy. On further questioning it became apparent that his staff were afraid that the newly bereaved relatives would break down. Throughout the social organization of death there are many 'private' rooms into which the bereaved next of kin are ushered.

Summary and conclusion

In this chapter I have focused on the survivor's response to the body as an object. The symbolic value of the decomposing corpse holds the key to understanding why we behave as we do when someone dies. In my study I wanted to explore the possibility that the dead body is 'matter out of place', dirty beyond its pathogenic potential. I was interested to see how our classification of the dead human body can be seen as reflecting the dominant ideologies of the time and how the polluting power of the corpse could be harnessed to generate control and authority. We can clearly see why the lack of a body to manipulate and to mourn over causes such consternation. We have been robbed of the very object with which we articulate our sacred and profane representations of death.

The corpse, human and yet non-human, has an ambiguity made even more threatening by its decay. The unfamiliar corpse is an object of both ritual and secular power. Classifying the cause of death, manipulating the appearance of the corpse, arresting its decay by embalming it and then destroying it altogether in the cremator are all attempts to gain human control over a natural event. The corpse's capacity to be used as a symbol system allows it to be harnessed to express many things, acting as a metaphor in this modern rational–scientific society, articulating traditional cultural norms, such as patriarchy, as well as playing out age-old beliefs regarding death and rebirth into the world of the ancestors. Yet our mastery is a mere illusion and the pretence is likely to break through at any moment. The ever-present danger of a collapse into chaos results in a rigorous application of various codes of conduct. This helps to explain the conservative nature of funerals.

The corpse is polluting and can contaminate those who come into contact with it. Harnessing our fears of the polluting power of the corpse, the deathwork professionals gain a great deal of control over their grieving clients who can easily be intimidated by the slightest mention of decay. The subtle way in which the funeral director can play on our pollution fears goes a long way to explain not only the spread of practices such as embalming, but also can account for our complete surrender of the disposal of the dead to deathwork professionals. Only the funeral director, embalmer and cremator attendant are equipped to care for the deteriorating corpse and the care of the cadaver takes place in specially designed 'backstage' areas. Another reason why the bereaved acquiesce in this is because they are in the process of disengaging from the corpse, turning their attention away from the decomposing body to the soul or spirit of the deceased. It is easy to imagine the soul as existing independently of the body. In their purely private realms the grieving relatives can develop a ghostly relationship with their dead's spirit. This may help to explain an apparently passive acceptance of the professionals' power and practices.

The professionals exact a price for taking care of the body. They in turn also pay a price. More than the bereaved, certain professionals become highly contaminated through their contact with the dead. Outside their place of work, they may resort to subterfuge to avoid admitting membership of a contaminated profession. The pollution of certain categories of deathwork professional is no accident. We have chosen to transfer the dirty work of disposing of our dead to a subgroup of workers and our fears of pollution regarding the corpse came before our distaste for this professional class. The bereaved friends and family may be contaminated by death, too, experiencing social and physical isolation in both the public and the private realms.

Contemporary mortuary practices seem to display many aspects of a rite of passage in which both the living and the dead go through a period of liminality, during which time they are transformed. Funerals bring families geographically and emotionally close. During this time family members try out their new roles within the family group. Certain sentimental items which belonged to the deceased are often informally dispersed well before the will has been read and the probate process completed. However much death has become a professional concern, it still poses age-old questions for the survivors. With the final ritual of reincorporation, which increasingly in British society is taking the form of a private rite in which the ashes are scattered or interred, the remains of the deceased are 'let go' into the domain of the dead. While this domain may not conform to religious scripture, this is a kind of afterlife. Indeed, in line with many other cultures' conceptualizations of the other world, the divide between the two can be a grey area. Ghosts and visitations were very a much a part of my respondents' experiences of having a husband on the other side.

6 Social representations of death

This is my greatest source of comfort. My husband's death was an excellent death. He was very happy . . . His friends, they liked him, too. They would say 'He is so interesting.' And you know, he just died without suffering. He had no illness. He would have hated . . . he was so impatient, he would be so unhappy. He wouldn't have been able to cope with, you know, long illness – psychologically. Nor was he romantic or a poet, but he did die like a poet. It was the best possible death for him. If it had happened ten years later it would have been better. But it has to be, this is the best way. This is how we would all like to go. He didn't suffer at all.

(Kate)

In any culture there are acceptable ways of talking about a death. For the Bolivian Laymi the time of death is peppered with talk about the stench of the body. Grieving family members who visit the deceased at the bedside talk about the stinking corpse. Harris notes that the same term of disgust is always used, (*wali th' 'usqa*), and she suggests that this custom of speaking in these terms serves some categorical, rather than descriptive or factual, purpose (1982: 50). It is not so much that the newly dead body really smells, but that using such an expression signifies that the person is dead (Harris 1982).

During my research I was forcibly struck by the frequency with which I was informed that deaths were good, bad, natural or unnatural. Drawing on my research findings I will argue that talking about death in these qualitative terms serves the same purpose in contemporary British culture as describing the corpse as smelling foul for the Laymi. These discourses about death, or 'narrative reconstructions', often make use of figures of speech or metaphors as expressive media (Radley 1994). These efforts to make sense of the world lie at the very foundations of our social constructions of life and death (see Berger and Luckmann 1967).

If the thought of chatting about the stinking corpse causes us to wince a little then we can appreciate the force with which these social norms operate. For every prescribed way of talking about death is balanced by the unacceptable and unthinkable. In contemporary British culture discussing the state of the corpse is taboo. A word search of the transcribed interview texts with the women revealed that the words 'corpse', 'cadaver', 'flesh', 'rotten', 'rot', 'decompose' and 'decay' were *never* used. Indeed, to a Western reader the mere suggestion that these grieving women might have used such words may seem offensive or naïve. But it is worth bearing in mind that the topic of these long conversations was the disposal of a body. In contrast, embalmers, funeral directors and coroners, who represent an exceptional group in our society, did not censor their corpse talk. The normal death etiquette does not apply to them. For these deathworkers the fact that the dead decompose was a 'normal' part of their working life. Thinking that this was the kind of information I was after and, quite possibly, challenging me for being nosy, I found their chat full of details about the sights, smells and even physical sensations of decay. I could never get used to this talk about the decomposition of the flesh and would catch myself recoiling in shock. It was a tremendous effort not to change the subject.

Talking about death

When lecturing on this topic to medical students and nurses doing masters degrees in palliative care I often ask them to share their ideas about good ways of dying. Faced by such a weighty question people are often thoughtful and creative. They imaginatively make use of various props to please the senses such as massage, flowers, music, scent and even drugs and alcohol. Usually their list will include dying without pain, dying surrounded by friends and dying in a state of preparation. There are also often contradictory descriptions of idealized death, such as sudden deaths. I can remember one man who immediately stated that he wanted to die in space. I presume that he did not intend his friends and family to be present.

I can remember giving a paper on the good death at a multi-disciplinary conference gloriously entitled 'Death, dying and disposal'. At question time a theologian asked me why I needed to talk about 'good' and 'bad' deaths. 'Are there not more interesting ways of thinking about death?' he asked. I think this question has merit, for the concept can seem oversimplified, a bit old fashioned, even stale. However much the insight that this process of dichotomization of the natural world into binary oppositions is arbitrary, this does not for a moment stop these representations from existing in lay consciousness. At the start of my research I did not set out to look at representations of the good or natural death: it was simply that if I was to listen to my respondents I had no choice but to talk about this concept.

Representations of death and of loss have undergone a process of dichotomization whereby dying and being bereaved are balanced between the desirable and the undesirable outcomes. It is often said that we do not know how to talk about death, but I would argue that we know only too well. We are almost blind to the fact that we are drawing on these representations of death. My underestimation of the importance of these representations at the early stages in the field is entirely consistent with their invisibility to me, a researcher undertaking own-culture research.

These are anything but profound categories in themselves for that is not their role. Saying a death is a good one is mainly a way of talking about it *as* good. It is not the content so much as the intent that is important here. For this reason attempting to take these descriptions at face value is doomed to failure as even the most cursory of analyses indicates that these representations are fluid and ever-changing. But however ordinary or even arbitrary these categories may appear it does not mean that they should not be taken seriously. Discourses about death reflect our ideologies and have an impact on what we do with the dead and how we treat the grieving. As I will show in the remaining chapters, the repercussions of labelling a death in these terms can be far-reaching.

An anthropological perspective of good deaths

Many cultures talk about the good death. Middleton (1982) describes the 'good' death of the Lugbara of Uganda. It is easy to see why this is seen as a fine way of leaving the world of the living. Here, Middleton describes the idealized death of a man.

> A man should die in his hut, lying on his bed, with his brothers and sons around him to hear his last words; he should die with his mind still alert and should be able to speak clearly even if only softly; he should die peacefully and with dignity, without bodily discomfort or disturbance; he should die at the time that he has for some days foreseen as the time of this death so that his sons and

brothers will be present; he should die loved and respected by his family. He should die physically when all these conditions have been or can be fulfilled and when he is expected to do so because he has said his last words and had them accepted by his kin and especially by his successor to his lineage status.

(Middleton 1982: 142)

The anthropologists Bloch and Parry (1982) argue that those groups who adhere to models of good deaths also tend to believe that these good deaths have some kind of regenerative potential. This can take the form of rebirth for the deceased – they die a good death and they are born into the afterlife – or for the group as a whole, in which good deaths are viewed as being good for the crops, the weather or for the as yet unborn members of the group.

> The 'good' death is thus the one which suggests some degree of mastery over the arbitrariness of the biological occurrence by replicating a prototype to which all such deaths conform, and which can therefore be seen as an instance of a general pattern necessary for the reproduction of life.
>
> (Bloch and Parry 1982: 15)

They argue that dying a 'good' death fits in with the very human desire to manipulate nature. One essential element in this discourse is the opposition of 'good' against 'bad'. We cannot have one without the other. 'Uncontrolled' or unpredictable deaths, such as those caused by accident or suicide, are viewed as 'bad' deaths and preclude the chance of regeneration, both for the deceased and the survivors. Indeed, bad deaths are very useful. They often befall those who do not behave well or those who belong to outgroups. The threat of dying a bad death acts as a warning to all and descriptions of horribly bad deaths are often entertained with some relish.

There may be negotiations and outright disagreements among the survivors as to whether a particular death was 'good' or 'bad' and this is part of the dialogue that surrounds a death. 'Good' deaths are therefore not automatic but are created through this discourse. Developing this theme of negotiation Bloch and Parry point to the subtle differences, first discussed by Durkheim in 1898, between negatively sanctioned suicide and positively sanctioned self-sacrifice. A social group which is at war is likely to promote the concept of a good death that befalls young, healthy men – a 'good' sacrifice. However, they point to the fact that sometimes there may be disagreement about which category, self-sacrifice or suicide, a death fits. For example, a hunger-striker's death could be viewed in different ways according to our political viewpoint.

Bloch and Parry (1982) note how funeral practices are, often, political events to do with the legitimation of authority. This explains the puzzling lack of funeral rites and the associated representations of 'good' or 'bad' death among hunter–gatherer groups, who have very simple social organizations. As Bloch and Parry point out, 'when there is no transcendental authority to be created the dead can be left alone' (1982: 42). This is a significant point. The representations of good and bad death are not psychological givens, expressed by individuals and shared between them, but culturally prescribed ways of viewing death which serve to delineate the social order.

Firth (1996) looked at British Hindu good deaths. These seem to fulfil many characteristics described by Bloch and Parry. Based on research which took place in southern England she explored the ways in which Hindus attempt to negotiate their ideal type of good death within the constraints of the institutional organization of death in this country.

> The ideal death is one in which a person dies in old age, having lived to see his or her grandson or great grandson. All unfinished business should have been dealt with regarding disposal of property (including gifts to charity); having arranged for the marriages of daughters or granddaughters; made amends for any quarrels; and said goodbye to members of the family.
>
> (Firth 1996: 97)

Firth is at pains to emphasize that the Hindu good death is not just about the organization of our secular affairs. The 'good death is set in the context of their entire lives, previous lives and the next life, and is thus part of a continuum of life, death and rebirth' (1996: 97). Preparations for the journey from the world of the living take the form of various dying rites, such as fasting, chanting God's name, imbibing sacred Ganges water and the leaf of the basil plant and choosing to die on the floor rather than on a bed. For the British Hindus in Firth's study, the worst possible fate was to die without being prepared. Bad deaths resulted in bad consequences. For example, she noted the distress caused to her respondents when essential dying rites, such as being at the bedside of the dying to hear their last words, chant sacred songs or administer sacred water, were blocked by hospital procedures. The repercussions of such bad deaths were extremely serious, spelling disaster for the surviving family who faced hauntings from a ghost capable of causing illness, bad luck, nightmares and infertility. Bad deaths can also befall those Hindus who die during certain phases of the moon. Such a death may indicate the future premature death of family members. In this instance it is possible to offset the danger by carrying out certain remedial rituals.

While Bloch and Parry are examining preindustrial and nonindustrial societies, they do briefly turn their attention to the industrialized West, noting that:

> In contemporary Western cultures the individual is given a transcendental value, the ideological stress is on his unique and *unrepeatable* biography, and he is conceived of in opposition to society and his death is therefore not a challenge to its continuity. Moreover, while man's nature may be seen as immutable, the existing social order is not. It is therefore not surprising that in this context the symbolic connection between death and fertility should be far more weakly stressed than it is in the cases we have considered here.
>
> (Bloch and Parry 1982: 15)

The links we make between death and fertility are much less clearly articulated and this undoubtedly has to do with the collective representation of the individual (see Farr 1998) and with the nature of contemporary Western societies. Further, British urban society is rather distanced from real deaths in the raw. Most urban people living in the Western world are singularly alienated from death. Although there are all-too-frequent periods of war, genocide, famine and epidemics, the sudden, unexpected and premature death of a loved one is not an everyday event. The disposal of the corpse has been handed over to professionals which has had the result of distancing the survivors from close contact with the deceased. In this context it makes sense that the ways in which we talk about death may be different. Yet I found that social representations of the good death abound. A number of people did see deaths in terms of rebirth and regeneration, although this was often in a rather individualized or personalized form. That people should still believe that their kin exist in the world of the dead should not surprise us. Many of the changes that have overtaken British society are relatively recent. For example, the mass exodus from church attendance barely spans a century. Further, various evangelical movements are making an impact on British society, particularly in the inner-city areas where I was doing my research.

Taking such things into consideration, ancient representations of death representing rebirth seem to be doing quite well.

Yet if the majority of people hold some kind of secular, non-regenerative representation of death as 'good' this begs the question as to what purpose these representations serve. Why do we continue to talk about a good death when most of us do not mean by that that the person died a death that was full of regenerative potential? Just as the 'alchemy' that links death with fertility (see p. 122) works to maintain the social order, current representations of death as 'good' because they were medically controlled or for that matter medically subversive are still about the attempt to gain control at this most disturbing and potentially chaotic moment in our life histories.

Contemporary British representations of death

During my fieldwork I was presented with many different, often contradictory, descriptions of good deaths. What is felt to have been 'good' for the deceased may not feel 'good' to the survivors, and vice versa. In contrast to the clearly articulated social mores of the past, dying well seems something of a free-for-all. We can die slowly, or fast, alone or in company and any of these types of dying may be described as a good death. How can we make sense of this diversity of contemporary 'good' deaths?

I have argued elsewhere (see Bradbury 1993a) that the good death had diversified into three 'types'. The ancient representation of the sacred good death has been largely overtaken by the modern medical good death which in turn is currently being challenged by the natural good death. These sacred, medical and natural good deaths, as 'ideal types', are rarely presented in pristine form in the real world. Yet I have found it useful to look at the source of our representations of death. If we look, we can discover where the factors used to describe good deaths come from; such insights may help us to find a way through the labyrinth of apparently contradictory statements and actions surrounding these idealized accounts. However, I do not want to imply by this any kind of linear development or progress towards the current state of play. These theoretical constructs are useful in explaining how our representations have changed over time although they should be conceptualized with an awareness that all three are still in regular use.

The sacred good death

> [My daughter] suddenly said, 'Are there any windows open?' This
> was about half-past eleven at night. And I said 'Why, are you
> hot?' and she said 'Oh, no, no, no, we must have a window open so
> that the spirit can go out.'
>
> (Eleanor)

Sebastian's death was 'perfect'. He died surrounded by his family, at
home. They played a recording of his favourite sonata for him and
opened a bottle of champagne to celebrate his well-lived life. He died
in his own bed, surrounded by love. Yet Eleanor freely admitted that
this beautiful death-bed scene was 'orchestrated' by her local hospital's
terminal support team who administrated high levels of opiates.
Counterpointing her description of this spiritual scene was her account
of what she felt was her husband's fight against death in the very last
moments of his life, as he thrashed and writhed about on the bed.

Margaret's husband also died of cancer and she too felt that, all
things considered, her husband's death was good. In her descriptions
of why the death was a good one she focuses on the 'death-bed scene'
in which the family gathered around the dying man in his private
room in their local hospital. She had a strong sense of his death
leading to his new life in heaven. Having eloquently described why
the death was good she then went on to say what was bad about the
death. Her husband seemed unaware that he was dying and he suffered
much pain, particularly when he was first admitted to hospital.

How are we to make sense of Eleanor's or Margaret's good deaths?
Ariès (1983), in his discussion of traditional attitudes towards death in
medieval Europe, suggests that such religious and commonplace
deaths were 'tamed'. In reality, it is highly unlikely that the experience
of dying or being bereaved was faced with anything like the kind of
calm acceptance or psychological health that, nostalgically, we like to
believe nowadays (Hockey 1996). Yet there seems to be evidence that
some people do face death calmly, believing that at death they will be
reborn. There are rare individuals who achieve this enviable state in
which their belief in rebirth allows them to let go of their life on earth.
More common than this great feat of acceptance is the faith of the
survivors that the deceased was reborn. For example, both Margaret
and Doris strongly believed that their husband's deaths were good
because, at death, they were reborn. However, in their accounts there
seemed to be little evidence that their husbands necessarily shared
their view.

In descriptions of the sacred death the death-bed scene plays a central role. The women would talk about the awareness—consciousness of their husband, his demeanour, the presence of family and friends, even the general setting (music, candles). These factors appear to draw on traditional images of dying the good death. Yet these were not medieval death-bed scenes but thoroughly modern affairs in which medical science played a leading role. Nowadays most religious people are perfectly happy to accept whatever medical care is available. The desperate struggle to resuscitate an individual who is supposed to be ready and prepared for death and the hereafter is not viewed by most of us as an inconsistency. The kind of complexity thrown up by the sharing of medical and sacred deaths is typical of the layered nature of our representations of death.

One important characteristic of the representations of the sacred good death is the way in which the death is seen as a social event. As was the case in the past, the contemporary sacred good death is viewed as a time to say goodbye to our loved ones. This social aspect extends beyond the immediate moment of death into the rituals that follow it. The shift in focus from the dying period to the grieving period makes sense if we consider that in a religious death the dead person's soul is still present and is open to communication during this period of ritual transition. The liminal soul can actually observe and perhaps even enjoy the mourning rituals of the bereaved.

> I think some of the most moving moments in my own work, my own ministry have been times when I have been at the bedside of a dying person and their family is with them and there is a recognition all around that this person is dying and that they can trust themselves to whatever lies beyond the moment of death. And there is a sadness, obviously . . . but there is also a willingness to face the future in confidence, [not] fear. So, basically, making a good death is about being aware of the experience, and accepting it rather than denying it.
>
> (The Reverend Ralph Peters)

Naturally, the clergy are active in promoting the sacred good death. But other professionals also make use of this representation. Think, for example, of Eleanor's orchestrated good death, described above. It is relatively easy to move between the representation of the medical good death, described in the next section, and the sacred good death. Once medical science has been proven to be incapable of saving or prolonging a life, the terminal support team can simply change tack. In this sense, the representation of the sacred good death takes on the character of a fancy-dress shop, a place where we can go to pick up costumes, although this is not to imply for a moment that these costumes do not serve important dramatic and spiritual purposes.

The medical good death

> The hospital was great . . . If we had paid a £1000.00 a day we couldn't have had better attention. The nurses and the doctors, too, we had a marvellous doctor. Our GP, Doctor Smith, he was super. . . They did everything they could.
>
> (Doris)

Doris did not feel prepared for her husband's death. She had not wanted to trouble the consultant and had failed to appreciate that Bert was dying. Yet despite the shock of realizing just a few days before his death that life would have to go on without him, she said that his death was a good one. Her explanation was focused on the medical care he received. Although this was through the NHS, it was the best that money could buy. It was clear that Bert's good medical death was well controlled by the medical personnel who looked after him. It appeared that he did not suffer pain and he was heavily sedated in the last few days of his life. Doris was quite unusual in her emphasis of the medical context of her husband's death. On the whole the women I spoke to drew on sacred or natural descriptions of why their husband's deaths were good or bad.

Medical staff and deathwork professionals, on the other hand, talked a great deal about idealized deaths that were good because they were medically controlled events. In a medical good death the physical act of dying is carefully orchestrated by medical personnel. Ideally the patient feels no pain and very often is unconscious. The medical good death does not necessarily have to be an expected event, however. They can be acute emergencies, in which all efforts are directed towards lifesaving activities.

Just as the sacred good death represented a way of controlling death through faith, the medical good death can also be viewed as a strategy for gaining control through the application of medical scientific knowledge. In this instance, the locus of control shifts from the dying person to those who take care of them. The focus is on the control of the physical symptoms of dying. For the medical personnel this kind of death is clearly easier to deal with than one that relies on the personal strength of character of the person who is dying. They are more likely to have a series of 'successful' deaths by using drugs than simply by hoping that the person will not experience and express great pain in the final stages of life. In the quotation below, the nurse is referring to the self-application of the Dimorphine syringe.

> We try and have the emphasis of letting the patient feel that they are in control of what's actually going on – until we get to a situation where they are unable to deal with it. And then we obviously have to step in for them.
>
> (Esther, nurse on surgical ward)

It is easy to see how medical science can increase the chances of having a 'good death'. For it not only allows us to control the behaviour of the dying person, but also facilitates control over the location and timing of the death. Controlling the timing of death reaches its logical conclusion in the unofficial euthanasia of terminally ill patients.

The natural process of dying is most obviously in human hands in intensive care units where life-support systems can be used as organs fail. Deaths in these conditions are highly stressful for staff and kin alike. In communicating with the relatives I found that staff drew upon the patient's heavily sedated and pain-free state. This was the only comfort they had to offer worried next of kin when the very definition of death can be blurred by technology. In the quotation below, John tells me how he talks to the relatives in such instances. Note the way in which he assumes that the unconscious state of the patient will comfort them. This kind of death is many miles away from the idealized social representation of the self-controlled and conscious sacred good death.

> We try and reinforce the feeling that they [the patient] don't know what is going on. The chances are that they don't know what is happening and that they aren't feeling any pain.
>
> (John, intensive care unit nurse)

Another instance in which the timing of a death appears to be in the hands of medical personnel is when doctors in intensive care units decide, with the family's permission, to switch off the life-support machine. Even if the person is already brain dead, the moment of switching off the machinery takes on a deadly significance.

If relatives are not present at the moment of death we find the description of death as painless to be the one most commonly sought after. This 'no pain' description of the medical good death becomes very familiar if we spend time in the presence of medical personnel or the bereaved. In the quotation below, it appeared that the very fact of medical intervention alone was enough to make a death 'good'. In this instance, the casualty doctor genuinely believed that the waiting relatives would feel better about the death if they thought the deceased received all the care and intervention available. An essential part of her 'breaking bad news' story was that 'we did everything we could'.

> I mean, quite often, if you bring them in and they are obviously dead you will actually wait ten minutes so the relatives actually think you have done something.
>
> (Charlotte, doctor)

> I would try and let them know what had happened and when the patient has been resuscitated I would say 'You know, the heart stopped and we tried to resuscitate using lots of drugs which are designed to get the heart going' and I would say that 'We were working for half-an-hour.'
>
> (John, intensive care unit nurse)

This was precisely the model that the patients' affairs officer worked on. In the next quotation she is talking about how she warns relatives that the clothing is cut or blood stained.

> When they brought him into casualty they tried to resuscitate and obviously they had to get to him as quickly as possible . . . so they cut the clothes . . . And they [the relatives] find that quite comforting actually . . . .To think that everything was done.
>
> (Trish, Patients' affairs officer)

What was particularly striking about these descriptions of the death was the lack of any description of the mental state of the dying patient or of the social context in which they died. Were they aware of what was happening to them? Did they make their peace with the world? Did they have time to pray? Were other family or friends present? Was a priest called? It is all too easy to see how questions of a social nature are deemed to be less important than the efforts to control the pain and symptoms of dying – or, for that matter, to save life.

Natural death and the natural good death

In a glorious tropical location Kate's husband drowned in her presence in a boating accident. Despite the horror of the event and the distress of observing her friends' desperate efforts to save his life, Kate thought there was a certain beauty to his death. She called her husband's good death 'natural'. She also mentioned that she drew comfort from the thought that it was quick and she contrasted it with those deaths that entail months of medical care, discomfort and pain.

In my small sample, I found that several different definitions of natural death appear to coexist in an extraordinary and often contradictory jumble. I came across two very different descriptions of a death in middle age, both called 'natural' by the next of kin. In contrast to Kate's husband's death at sea, Ann's husband died quietly at home after weeks of care in which his impending demise was openly acknowledged. Kate felt her husband's death by drowning was natural simply because he died 'in nature', 'by nature'. Ann's husband's death acquired a naturalness in her eyes because of their mutual preparation for the event.

Death is a natural event so one would think that it would be logical to describe any death in this way. Yet calling a death 'natural' is no simple matter. This is a representation that is loaded with meaning and constantly changing. To a large extent, the very definition of 'natural' lies in the eyes of the beholder. We may mean many different things when we talk of a natural death. In this context, it is all too easy to see how there may be disagreement. Indeed, issues of naturalness often lie at the heart of debates such as the one currently raging around assisted euthanasia.

Prior (1989), in a discussion of the natural death, points to the surprising fact that the law has never distinguished between the categories of 'natural' and 'unnatural death'. Having considered the fluid nature of this term, this comes as no great surprise. Perhaps it is useful to quote him here.

> The Coroners Rules of 1953 contained a number of recommendations for verdicts, and we can perhaps glean something of the meaning of the terms natural and unnatural from the verdict categories. Fourteen verdicts are listed: Murder, Manslaughter, Infanticide, Killed himself, Attempted or self-induced abortion, Accident/Misadventure, Execution of sentence of death, Justifiable or excusable homicide, Natural causes, Industrial disease, Want of attention at birth, Chronic alcoholism/addiction to drugs,

Aggravated by lack of care/self-neglect and Open. And, as one can see, this pot-pourri of socio-legal and medico-legal distinctions contains a great many overlaps and ambiguities, not least of which are those contained in the term 'natural causes'.

(Prior 1989: 51)

The definitions of naturalness and unnaturalness used by a coroner are confined to a narrow band of professionals: lawyers, the registrar and the police. Other professionals involved with the same death will quite possibly label it more conventionally, in spiritual or medical terms. Isolated in a medico-legal ivory tower, the coroner and his associates balance the causes of death in their own unique way. While I was talking to a barrister even she admitted that she would have to go and look up the definition for 'natural causes'. As far as the coroner and registrar are concerned, deaths by natural causes are not bad because they do not imply negligence or foul play. Yet being 'not bad' does not necessarily mean 'good'. The death is simply 'natural'. On the other hand, the badness implied by an 'unnatural' death has a huge impact on the relatives of the deceased. A death thus categorized immediately flings the survivors into questions of causation. For example, a death that friends and family may have labelled as a medically good death, however shocking or unexpected, may be put under threat by the thought that, say, medical malpractice led to the death; things could have been done differently; the deceased may have survived. Further, a death labelled as due to unnatural causes often leads to further investigations. Then the coroner's physical possession of the corpse, and the things that are done to that corpse during a post-mortem, make their control, and thus their definition of a death, indisputable. Negotiation is out of the question.

By the eighteenth century the ancient view of natural death as part of life's pattern had been overtaken by a new concern to control the process of dying with medical remedies (Hockey 1990). People were now trying to negotiate with death and as a result their conceptions of its naturalness were shifting. Already, deaths represented medical defeats. By the twentieth century death was conceived in terms of disease and disease management (Hockey 1990). In a society for whom the deaths of even the very elderly is seen in terms of the progression of a variety of diseases, it is easy to see that there is little space for a view of death as natural. Most deaths are 'failures'. In Illich's (1976) analysis of the natural death he charts the gradual demise of the concept that he suggests is linked to the rise to power of the medical sciences in the West.

The medicalisation of society has brought the epoch of the natural death to an end. Western man has lost the right to preside at his act of dying.

(Illich 1976: 207)

In its place stands the good death that was 'that of the standard consumer of medical care' (Illich 1976: 198). The bad death, in contrast, is the death that took place without any kind of treatment, a domain of the disordered, unpredictable and uncontrolled (Hockey 1990). Thus what was natural became bad.

The quotation from Illich, above, was written in the mid-1970s and much has changed since then. I found that some people believed that a death was 'good' because it was 'natural'. It appears the natural death as 'good' is back on the scene. If the essential ingredient of any good death is the sense of control, what gives us that feeling of being in control in these cases? I would suggest that these good natural deaths were good because they represented a break from what has increasingly been seen as the overbearing and intrusive medical control of the dying.

In the past life was short and liable to end with a relatively brief period of illness, caused by what would now be regarded as an easily curable infection. Such deaths usually allowed for some kind of preparation, but not a long wait. Contemporary deathways are very different. Morgan (1995) notes that at the end of the twentieth century most people expect a long lifespan ending after a possibly long period of suffering from a chronic debilitative disease. Expanding on this theme, Walter (1994), in his discussion of what he calls 'neo-modern' deaths, notes that with medical developments we now often have time to contemplate our fate during a protracted period of dying. In this environment the treatment of the dying person has been turned into something of a craft. Herein lies the locus of control.

Many dying people are better informed medically because they now have time to be. If the traditional human condition is that of living with death, and the modern condition one of death denied, the post-modern condition is more one of living with dying.

(Walter 1996: 198)

A typical example of this rebellion against modern medical interventions is provided by the natural death movement. This movement was launched in the early 1990s in a flurry of media attention. Drawing loosely on the natural birth movement of the 1970s (Leboyer 1975),

which argued for the rights of women to give birth without unnecessary and intrusive medical interventions, the natural death movement
is concerned for the rights of the dying. Focusing in particular on
diagnosed terminal conditions, such as cancer, the natural death centre
offers helpful and practical advice on alternative pain relief, 'home
deaths' and 'living wills' (Albery *et al.* 1993). As far as possible, the
dying are encouraged to take control of their deaths and to reject a
passive, 'patient' role. This movement has much in common with the
hospice movement. No one is suggesting that people should die
without any kind of pain relief or intervention: merely that they
should retain some sense of dignity, personhood and self-determination. This would appear to reflect a postmodern habitat where, Bauman argues, individuals are encouraged to embrace 'DIY operations'
(Bauman 1992b: 194) such as jogging, dieting and slimming. In this
instance it is DIY dying.

At first glance, the natural death movement's criteria are much like
the sacred good death's. Both are based on expected deaths. However,
there is one profound difference. The natural death advocate is not
expected to call for a priest or necessarily believe in immortality
although themes of regeneration are thoroughly aired with a tour of
the world's religions in the 'natural death handbook'. Dying the
natural death movement's good death seems to be primarily about
honouring the individuality and personality of the dying person.

The empowerment of the consumer continues after death as the
survivors are encouraged to take an active role in the disposal of the
deceased. The movement gives information about how to carry out a
'do-it-yourself funeral' including much advice on skills such as laying-
out the dead at home and how to make one's own coffin. Funeral
directors' fees come under strong criticism, as does the practice of
unnecessary embalming. Thus this 'natural' death is not only to be
freed from the medical profession but also from the funeral trade.

Advocating the use of recycled cardboard coffins, cotton shrouds and
'woods for the dead' and rejecting the wasteful use of timber, plastics,
fabric and embalming fluids we can see how the movement became
associated with the green movement. Yet, perversely, with its detailed
and scientific talk regarding how to compost our dead, Hockey (1996)
notes that the natural death movement is involved in a delicate
balancing act in which it wavers precariously between a discourse
concerning 'nature' and one concerning 'science'. In his analysis of
the term 'natural', Elias points to the romantic vision of nature as an
idealized escape from the modernizing world. In such a vision 'it is
supposed that everything she does, everything that is "natural", must

be good and salutary for human beings' (Elias 1985: 79). He adds menacingly: '"Nature" has no intentions; it knows no goals; it is entirely purposeless' (1985: 80). The Cartesian opposition, in which nature is put in opposition to science, permeates the natural death movement. Thus natural deaths are natural not so much because they happen randomly or purposelessly but because they reject what is conceived of as the 'unnatural' world of medical science.

There is yet another type of natural good death. This is the sudden and unexpected death that leaves no time for preparation, disease, pain or farewells. While it is questionable how many people really want to die with no warning, it is still true that people talk about this as a kind of good death, both as an ideal for themselves and as a justification of a 'good' label for the death of their loved ones. Like the medical death and the slow natural death, this sudden 'natural' death would also appear to be profane. In a culture that has become unfamiliar with pain, it is possible that this sudden natural death is popular precisely because it precludes the chance of suffering. Thus those people who claim to want such a sudden death, such as the medical student who stated that he wanted to die suddenly in space, are probably referring to the painlessness of these unexpected deaths. They are touching the medical model of the pain-free death that first arose in the Victorian era. For our predecessors such deaths would be the epitome of a bad death (Ariès 1983).

Making the death good

These descriptions of the contemporary good death may leave us with the impression that the choice of a label is totally arbitrary, a sort of morbid free-for-all whereby we can have no expectation of consensus or consistency. This is not actually the case. There are common-sense features of a good death that are relatively easy to identify. These factors are very similar to those found in other cultures. My data analysis revealed several features which were found to be particularly important to my sample of respondents at the time that I was interviewing them. It is quite possible that the very women I spoke to may describe their husband's deaths differently now. While these are not necessarily the only ingredients in a good death recipe, it is useful to look at them. In doing so we clearly see how a long dying trajectory can 'set' the scene for the label of the good death.

Based on my data, the women interviewed described the following as the most important factors which contributed to a good death: a) both parties having an awareness of the dying period; b) both husband

and wife being prepared for the death; c) having pain under control; d) the wife being present at the moment of death; and e) for some, being at home for the death. Kellehear (1990), who worked with patients dying with cancer, Samerel (1995) who studied nurses' perceptions of a good death and Weisman (1978) have also compiled strikingly similar lists of features.

My respondents also talked of the positive factors of dying without protracted illness, without suffering the ills of a long old age and dying with dignity. These rationalizations were often added on to the end of their discussions of why deaths were good.

> It was a good death, for Ken. A brilliant death for Ken. Because Ken hated illness. He couldn't stand it.
>
> (Paula)

An awareness of dying was found to be an important consideration when the widows came to categorize their loved one's death as good. Both Ann and Eleanor made the most of the last months of their husbands' lives. Although belonging to a state of 'open awareness' should not be presumed to imply that it was easy to talk to their husbands about their impending death, it did give them the chance to express themselves. In contrast Bert was kept in ignorance about his condition. In the last days, care was taken not to raise his suspicions, which at times entailed white lies to explain his daughter's presence at his bedside.

The sense of 'being prepared' is highly subjective. Being prepared does not simply mean being told by a medical practitioner that our loved one will die, but rather on the self-reflective awareness that death is imminent. We do not necessarily feel more prepared for a death when we are elderly or if we have been married for many decades. For example, Beth's husband was 84 when he died and she described his death as a complete surprise. Being prepared increases the likelihood of being present at the death and gives time to create a good death environment. We can say our goodbyes, organize our material affairs and muster resources for the death bed. It is still possible to have a good death even if we were not prepared. By referring to the medical model of the painless good death, a sudden death that precludes the experience of pain can be elevated to the status of a natural good death.

Naturally, the painlessness of their husbands' deaths was of paramount importance to the women. This was a source of comfort. Descriptions of the death bed often centred around details of pain relief. Painlessness can arise from two factors: drug regimes or the suddenness of the death. Janet's husband died of a heart attack during his sleep. Janet was greatly comforted when the coroner told her that her husband would have felt no pain.

> To see him, he was still asleep. He hadn't even moved. I mean, if he had been in pain he would have called out. I would have heard him.
>
> (Janet)

Those women who were in attendance at the time of death thought that their presence was a crucial feature of their husband's good death. There was a certain confidence in their tone as they discussed who was there, the mood at the death bed and details of the physical death itself. This is apparent in the descriptions given by Margaret (see p. 147) and by Sarah. Margaret and the children gathered around the dying man. Everyone had felt very involved in the dying period and his death was, in some ways, rather beautiful. In contrast, Ruth felt the fact she had not been with her husband when he died in the street was the reason his death was bad. She worried about his last moments. Had he been in pain? Did he ask for help? In an effort to put her fears to rest she reconstructed his last movements that morning, visiting the bank where he had deposited some money. She even looked at his signature to see if it looked shaky.

Although most people die in hospital, dying at home continues to be a popular option. The women were aware of the advantages of maintaining a degree of control over the manner of their husband's death. For Ann, who cared for her husband throughout his illness, death at home was cited as the most important reason for it being a good death.

> It was at home. That is probably the most important, so he was able to spend the last weeks, when he knew he was getting worse, he didn't have to face leaving home.
>
> (Ann)

> I was pleased he was home where he wanted to be. With his own things. Well, we haven't got a lot. But he was home.
>
> (Christine)

They also talked about the advantages of being able to spend time with the body before the funeral director removed it.

Institutionalized death was talked about in almost universally critical terms. The women talked of the strain of meeting new people, of adapting to the hospital routine and visiting hours, and of difficulties in relaxing or feeling a sense of privacy. While Margaret felt the staff had been fantastic during her husband's illness, she was confused and hurt by their behaviour after her husband's death. She felt she had been pushed out of the ward (see p. 59).

The bad deaths

When he left here (for the hospital) he was in very good health, it seemed to me. They just wanted him in for a couple of days for tests, they said. I thought, 'Well, that will be a week, it always is.' But I didn't think he was going to die, I certainly didn't think that. And we might have planned things rather different if we had realized that he was going to die, or if there was a possibility. Because we never talked about death.

(Beth)

Despite the social pressure to present the death as a good event, some deaths are bad. Beth regretted that her husband, Keith, seemed to be in pain and she was saddened by the fact that they never had a chance to say their farewells. When Beth's husband took a turn for the worse she decided not to tell him that he was gravely ill. Her husband's lack of awareness of his closeness to death and the sadness she felt that prior to his days of unconsciousness she was not able to say goodbye to him were the chief reasons why she said she felt his death was bad. Christine's husband had lung cancer. Failing fast, he died within weeks of the first diagnosis. He died in Christine's presence, at home. They received the help of a terminal support team and Keith was given large doses of pain killer. Although this death had the potential to be sculpted into some kind of medical good death, the personal circumstances of this couple were such as to make this outcome unlikely. Poor, ill and socially isolated Christine was not interested in polite presentations of suffering. She was angry with her husband's consultant who changed his prognosis. Christine said that there was no way in which she could call her husband's death good: 'There was nothing good about it.'

There are types of death so violent and so generally unpleasant that any observer would describe the death as a bad one. Naturally, in these instances there is no social pressure to hide fury and upset and the bereaved next of kin are free to describe the death as bad. Ruth's husband died while out shopping. Unfortunately, this was during an ambulance-workers' strike. A passer-by valiantly attempted to give the dying man heart massage and mouth-to-mouth resuscitation. But by the time the army ambulance arrived, half-an-hour later, Ruth's husband was dead. That Ruth called her husband's death a bad one comes as no surprise.

However, even in violent deaths we may succumb to the pressure of presenting a death as good. Susan's husband was killed in a car accident. Susan was abroad at the time. In the first phase of our interview I had no doubt that this was a bad death and was therefore surprised when she said that the death was good. The next day, Susan phoned me. She was troubled by her description of the death; she wanted to say that she really felt it was a bad death. In the artificial environment of our interview, in which the hidden agenda appears to have been the state of Susan's mental health, she had succumbed to the pressure to pretend that the death was good, when she really felt the reverse.

Whatever the circumstances surrounding a bad death, it is characterized by a sense of lacking control. The timing and the suddenness of the death are crucial factors. Some deaths are nearly always viewed as bad by professionals and bereaved alike: for example, deaths resulting from car crashes, murders, suicides, accidents, cot deaths, drug addiction and mass deaths (such as fires and explosions in public sites, 'crushes' in crowds). As far as deathworkers are concerned, bad deaths are highly salient. They are upsetting and memorable. Other deaths are more ambiguous and open to negotiation. For example, a funeral director may view the death of a child as bad, while the child's family may feel that while words could not describe their anguish, the actual moment when their child died was 'good'.

Summary and conclusion

> He was in the kitchen, and I walked down, and he took me in his arms and he said 'I have got cancer of the bowel, and I can't be operated, and I don't know how long I have got to live.' So what I said at that point, this was quite some time before his death, of course. 'Oh dear,' I said. 'If that is so, we will just have to do the best we can, and get through it together.'
>
> (Ann)

It may sound quite strange if someone said 'It was a good death because he died of cancer' yet the cause of death is the single most important factor in influencing the categorization of a death. It is precisely the cause of death that determines factors such as awareness levels, site of death and the degree of pain felt. This is not just another example of the primacy of the medical model, for the mode of death probably influences the classification of a death for anyone in any culture. However, the predictability of the disease type is of particular importance in our industrialized culture. If medical personnel can help orchestrate the moment of death, for example by sending the dying patient home for an old-fashioned death-bed scene that is carefully planned with the use of pain-killing drugs, then the surviving family is more likely to say that the death was a good one. I am not suggesting that cancer is necessarily a good way to die. I am simply arguing that the cancer-type death provides us with the optimal conditions for controlling and manipulating the process of dying and the death itself which, in turn, gives everyone the right mix of factors by which to justify the death as good.

This does not mean that less-controlled deaths will not be called good as well. In an environment where the painlessness of a death has become a key factor (reflecting as it does a triumph of medical science) then the painlessness of death through its very suddenness may mean it, too, qualifies for a 'good' category. Alternatively, the survivors may not feel the need to call the death a good one, although all the factors that would make the death a good one may be in place. Christine felt her husband's death was 'bad' even though Keith's death appears to represent an 'ideal' cancer death.

Current talk about death appears to cluster around the relative 'goodness' or 'naturalness' of the event. Drawing on their own idiosyncratic world views, people construct a variety of good deaths using a selection of representations of death, mixing and matching according to the context of the death. Bloch and Parry (1982) outlined the importance of controlling the location and timing of a death in order to create an illusion of human power. In a modern Western context one way of gaining maximum control of a dying person is through intensive medical intervention. Leaving alone the acts of suicide and murder which have always been possible, contemporary Western cultures have the means to orchestrate deaths to an extraordinary degree, thereby creating the 'medical good death'. Meanwhile the 'natural good death', apparently a radical new representation, proves to be anchored in other anti-medical movements, such as the natural birth movement. The third representation of the good death, the 'sacred good death', continues to exist. These good deaths are counterbalanced by lurid descriptions of nasty deaths. However shocking bad deaths may be, we appear to have an avid interest in them. Excepting the deaths of celebrities, just about every death reported in the media is 'bad'; we play out the opposition between good and bad by focusing on the latter and in the process we articulate the good ideal death.

I have been emphasizing that different representations are used simultaneously, thereby making it impossible to construct any kind of time-boundary between the different types. It is for this reason that in the labels I have applied to these ideal types I have consciously tried to avoid the suggestion of a linear development of any kind. Contemporary, postmodern deaths *include* representations of the sacred and medical good death and are not just a development from them or a reaction against them.

This contradictory mix of representations is typical of the kind of postmodernist discourse described by Bauman (1992b). Indeed, labelling another person's death as good or bad seems to be full of those aspects of ambivalence and contingency that Bauman (1992b) describes as features of the postmodern condition. Billig (1992) has highlighted the argumentative nature of talk. The representations I identified during my time with the doctor, nurse, coroner, registrar, funeral director, cremator attendant, memorial counsellor and grieving next of kin were far from uniform. Their definitions were neither stable nor consistent. Within the same sentence people would shift between different representations as they bounced ideas off me, thus presenting me with an ever-changing kaleidoscope of various types of goodness and of the play between good and bad factors.

These representations are not social facts. They do nevertheless have an impact on our experience of the physical world. At the beginning of the chapter I discussed the ways in which the medical students and nurses found it easy to articulate their ideas about a good death. Whatever the representation used by the deathwork professional, it is not too difficult to discover the motive. Providing that the death is not indisputedly bad, calling other people's deaths 'good' may be a simple way of coping with the stress of an extraordinary job. The labelling of a death is also contingent on the perceived social value of the person who is dying. The physical deaths of those who have already suffered a social death are unremarked events, in which a discourse regarding the relative merits of that person's death is not deemed necessary.

Although politically correct rhetoric may emphasize the need for the dying person's self-determination (Samerel 1995), these social representations of death are prescriptive. Consequently, in many cases, contemporary representations of the good death continue to serve the purpose of the legitimization of medical authority. In a context in which many aspects of the disposal of our dead has been appropriated by small businesses, the representation of the good death is easily harnessed into the job of keeping the grieving customer compliant. Thus it is that the family visiting the funeral parlour's chapel of remembrance find themselves in the extraordinary position of praising the embalmer's efforts to create the reposeful, but still very dead, relative. In this sense, the undertaker's habit of 'directing their expectations upwards' (see p. 81) seems less quaint.

7 Social representations of loss

> I came straight back here after he died. When the curate, you know, asked me what to do I said 'I am going straight back home.' And I did, and, I sort of, you know, sort of gritted my teeth, opened the door, and went to bed. And, er, I have been here ever since.
>
> (Beth)

In Chapter 1 I discussed how psychology became separated from its parent discipline of philosophy early on in its career. Keen to affiliate itself to the natural sciences the fledgling discipline whole-heartedly embraced the quest of discovering the natural laws that lay behind human behaviour and thought. Part of this package of positivism was the adoption of quantitative methodologies.

Stimulated by the mass bereavements caused by the two World Wars, the topic of grief has proved to be very attractive to psychologists since the 1940s. The emotional and physiological repercussions of loss and of bereavement became the focus of study. In many ways the 'discovery' that the emotion of grief could be likened to a disease represented a shining example of the modern future of psychology. The social nature of bereavement was neglected. While Durkheim and Hertz had both argued that apparently individual acts, such as suicide or grief, could be culturally manufactured, their sociological theories of emotion were ignored. In the late 1980s, while studying for an introductory diploma in social psychology, having just graduated with an anthropology degree, I was introduced to the various depression and stress models of grief. I was stunned to come across this image of grief. The gulf between my anthropologically inspired conception of loss as an essentially social phenomenon and the psychological models of grief as individual experience open to pathology seemed insurmountable, as I still believe they are. In this chapter I briefly review the development of the medical models of grief. The dichotomisation of grief into healthy and unhealthy outcomes demonstrates, once again, the powerful impulse to split the natural world into binary oppositions.

Presenting grief as disease

The psychiatric and psychological literature on bereavement confirms the claims of sociologists that death has become medicalized in modern societies (Charmaz 1980; Glaser and Strauss 1968; Littlewood 1993; Prior 1989; Sudnow 1967). We not only die within the medical model of health and disease, we grieve within it too. Talk of 'outcomes', either healthy or pathological, and the associated 'symptoms' of loss leave us with the distinct impression that grief is a disease rather than a universal experience. The pathologization of grief is a symptom of its individualization. By situating grief in the sick mind and body of the individual we can then exercise our predilection for blaming the individual for personal misfortune (Heider 1958).

The psychiatrist Lindemann (1944) was the first to suggest that grief could be viewed as a syndrome with somatic distress and psychological trauma. His notion that people had 'grief-work' to be done was soon followed by other studies which aimed to trace the symptomatology of grief (Bowlby 1981; Clayton 1979, Clayton *et al*. 1968; Engel 1961; Parkes 1965, 1986). By the late 1960s, Maddison and Viola (1968) could compile a list of all the symptoms so far identified, as if they were compiling a diagnostic list of symptoms for a medical textbook. Various psychometric measures of grief were developed such as the 'Texas Inventory of Grief' (Faschingbauer *et al*. 1977; Zisook *et al*. 1982). Comprehensive summaries of and discussions about these studies can be found in Stroebe and Stroebe (1987) and Rando (1995).

Great interest also focused on the ways in which these 'symptoms' could be seen to proceed in phases (Bowlby 1981; Clayton *et al*. 1968; Parkes 1965). Thus we could observe 'shock' as being a characteristic of early grief and 'depression' as one of later grief. Stroebe and Stroebe (1987) note that several different models of the stages and phases of grief have been developed over the years but there is general agreement about the character of this process. Individuals were viewed to proceed through a series of stages such as numbness, followed by yearning and protest, despair and, finally, recovery and restitution (Bowlby 1961, 1971, 1975, 1981; Glick *et al*. 1974). Despite the acknowledgement that people actually do not necessarily proceed through the phases of grief in an orderly manner and that they may, indeed, skip phases altogether (Stroebe and Stroebe 1987), this was a point which has often been overlooked. The model proved to be very seductive.

Stroebe and Stroebe (1987) argue that the detailed description of 'normal' grief was seen as necessary in order to define abnormality. From the start the balance between healthy and pathological grief was established. Pathological grief was conceptualized as grief gone wrong. Once again, it was Lindemann (1944) whose empirical study of morbid grief set the stage for a fashion in research that lasted several decades. Lindemann suggested that delayed grief, in which the bereaved person faced their loss with apparent cheerfulness (Stroebe and Stroebe 1987), was the most common form of pathological grief. Clearly influenced by Freud (1957, first published in 1917), Lindemann argued that the delaying of grief led to certain distortions, such as overactivity. Healthy grief, in contrast, was that which was worked through. Following on the heels of this study, Parkes (1964a, 1965) identified three major forms of pathological grief: namely, chronic, delayed and inhibited. Once again, this stimulated further research in the field (Volkan 1970), and notably the work of Parkes and Weiss (1983) who reformulated the classification of pathological grief. Thus the types became unexpected grief syndrome, ambivalent grief syndrome and chronic grief syndrome (Stroebe and Stroebe 1987).

In the early pioneering studies of grief as disease, the reader rarely got to hear what the bereaved had to say. Either the data were not based on the speech of the bereaved at all, relying instead on questionnaire responses, or the speech of the respondent was weeded out in the creation of a 'scientific' text for a journal or book. I suggest that the object of study was not the self-reflective person who had suffered a loss, but the representation of grief as some kind of malaise. In this sense the search for the symptomatology of grief became a self-fulfilling prophesy. It is of note that these silenced voices are, in the main, those of women. Given the longevity of women, the majority of research on grief and bereavement has been based on widows. In this context, the pathologization of grief takes on a sinister hue. It is probably not too outlandish to suggest that we are accessing a sexist discourse about women and their potentially unhealthy reactions to psychological trauma (see Showalter 1987).

The 'vulnerability' factors

Having identified the two different paths we could take on suffering a loss and the associated symptoms we are likely to exhibit, the question arose as to why people respond in these different ways. The answer was thought to be found in personality variables but, as Stroebe and Stroebe (1987) point out, these studies have proven to be inconclusive (Parkes and Weiss 1983). It was necessary, therefore, to look at other possible reasons for the differences in reactions between individuals: namely, their biographies and the context of their grief. Not surprisingly, these biographies proved to be social histories. The positivist, individualized and medical perspectives on grief had to come to terms with the social aspects of bereavement. These social descriptions have been lumped together with a few 'individual' features, such as age at bereavement, and are usually called 'vulnerability' or 'risk' factors. The rationale for these titles is that the more factors that are weighing against us, the more vulnerable to an adverse grief reaction we become. They have attracted a huge amount of research (Ball 1977; Cain 1972; Clayton *et al.* 1973; Lundin 1984a, 1984b; Maddison and Walker 1967; Parkes 1970, 1975; Sanders 1981, 1983). The nine vulnerability factors commonly cited are: 1) pre-existing relationship with deceased; 2) type of death; 3) the response of family and social network; 4) concurrent stress or crisis; 5) age of bereaved; 6) sex of bereaved; 7) class of bereaved; 8) religiosity; and 9) the personality of the bereaved (Stroebe and Stroebe 1987).

This list seems to describe the 'culture' or 'society' within which the bereaved person lives. Radley (1994), in his critique of stress and vulnerability, argues that the very concept of 'stress' can be viewed as a social representation. Further, we find that even the apparently 'individual' characteristics of the age and gender of the grieving person are, to a certain extent, socially constructed phenomena (see Caplan 1987). For example, Strauss and Howe (1991) argue that social scientists need to understand generational differences before they make generalizations regarding the attitudes and values of any social group; the differences in experience between the elderly and the young go beyond the issue of age as they also reflect the social and historical context of people's lives.

There is a vast literature concerned with the interaction between the various 'vulnerability factors'. An excellent review of the literature can be found in Stroebe and Stroebe (1987). Concerned with 'verification', these factors are often described in terms of operational definitions before being isolated from other variables. Thus for example, in a controlled study, Sanders (1980), concerned with the influence of 'religiosity' on outcome, compared people's church-attendance rates with various grief-experience inventories. The gap between going to church and having faith may be large indeed. I have difficulty in recognizing the vivid experience of culture in these reductionist descriptions of behaviour.

Within the psychiatric tradition of research on grief, there are some authors who have attempted to incorporate the social while adhering to a positivistic view that rational organization, or 'natural laws', characterize the human condition (Amir and Sharon 1982; Lopata 1973a, 1973b, 1979; Parkes 1975; Raphael 1984; Stroebe and Stroebe 1987). In many ways these books and articles do redress the balance. For example, Stroebe and Stroebe review the findings and debates between those who believe that emotion, such as grief, can be viewed as physiologically driven and those who view it as shaped by culture. Yet while Stroebe and Stroebe argue that it is more useful to take the middle ground – one that accepts that emotional experiences are shaped by both distinct bodily reactions and by social norms – their rigorous preference for positivist research techniques suggests that any synthesis would be an uneasy one. Meanwhile, all too often, ethnographic material from other cultures is implicitly criticized from within this positivist framework. In the same volume Stroebe and Stroebe (1987) review anthropological studies concerning grief and the impact of bereavement rituals before bemoaning the lack of proper empirical studies (1987: 51).

An academic field in crisis

Identifying grief as a syndrome was a highly satisfying activity. Such labelling and categorizations offers some feeling of control over the disorderly nature of grief. As the field became established, students were introduced to the topic as a scientific fact. As D. J. Davies (1996) notes, this may have been particularly attractive to those young adults who, owing to changing patterns of mortality, had little experience of bereavement.

While authors such as Stroebe and Stroebe were at pains to emphasize that the phasic model should not be viewed as 'normative prescriptions' (1987: 16), such is the manner in which 'science' gets communicated to the lay population that there was never much hope that their provisos would be heard. With the dissemination of the stage–phase model into the popular culture via the mass media, the idea that we do not necessarily have to go through all stages was lost.

Hockey (1990) notes that, in the early 1970s, the study of grief began to undergo subtle changes as a response to developments in the hospice movement. Just as the experience of dying had undergone a revolution, now the grieving next of kin also began to find a voice (Parkes 1986; Worden 1991). In 1984, Raphael's fine study of bereavement, published in handbook format, broke many of the traditions set up over the previous four decades. She illustrated her descriptions of loss using case studies. Many other books followed on the trail of this release during a period in which research findings, previously confined to journals, found their way into books for the general public and caring professions (Boston and Trezise 1987; Johnson 1987; Sanders 1989; Wilcox and Sutton 1985; Worden 1991). Many of these stage–phase models of grief are, essentially, reformulations of the medical model of grief in which 'good' desirable outcomes are balanced against pathological outcomes. In America a tradition of research which utilizes the concept of 'grief work' in the name of psychological health remains popular. For example, Rando suggests that 'these are the processes that the mourner must success-fully complete in order to accommodate the loss in a healthy manner' (1995: 221).

Recently, interest in the description of the grief reaction has waned and the flood of publications has reduced to a trickle. Recent critiques of this position, largely to be found in sociological volumes, abound (Charmaz 1980; Cleiren 1991; Davies 1997; Hockey 1990; Prior 1989). In retrospect it is clear that the psychiatric and psychological research into the grief reaction reached an impasse similar to the crisis within social psychology in the early 1970s when Rosenthal's (1966) 'experimenter effects' and Orne's (1952) 'demand characteristics' exposed the social nature of the laboratory. Despite the desire to remove the social factors of bereavement and to facilitate the focus on those all-important individual differences, the social has intruded, spoiling our individualistic conception of grief as disease. Within its confines the traditional study of grief and bereavement from the perspective of the medical model became not just unfashionable: it became unresearchable.

The reductionist model of grief has had a great impact on the bereavements of British and American people during the late modern era. As Hockey (1990) notes, the very nature of grief – suffering – is neither preventable nor treatable and as a result it is distanced and avoided. Traditionally, hearing about the pain of loss was part of the pastoral care provided by the priest. In times when science and the expert were enjoying ascendancy, the diagnosis of medical conditions gave health professionals something to do when faced with a patient or client in grief. The grieving were handed over to personnel whose response to their loss was, all too often, to supply drugs for depression.

While acknowledging that in some people bereavement does spark off psychopathological states or severe physiological reactions, we can see that, thanks to the expectations of GPs and other health-care professionals, people come to experience their loss as a medical 'condition' which needs to be overcome.

> She said, 'It will take a year, I think. That's what I think, it will take a year.' I remember being outraged. I almost said to her 'You bloody try it, Maria.'
>
> (Susan)

The conception took root in British and American society that we could 'recover' from grief. This has had many, many repercussions. In the quotation given below, Janet is describing her first visit to her GP since her bereavement.

> He did say to me 'You still get upset don't you?', as if it was odd. After eight months, you still get upset. And as I said to him, 'It is hard, we were fifteen when we were first together'. 'It is a long time.' And I looked at him, and he just grinned, and I almost said to him, 'Well, perhaps you two don't get on so well.' Well, I mean, me and my husband was fighting . . . like cat and dog sometimes, we weren't lovey-dovey. But you still miss them through those ups and downs you had, you know what I mean? You still miss all that. You know. Your nagging, and all that, and the door slamming. You know, after 42 years, all those years, you just. You know. [The doctor's] attitude to me was just 'Eight months, you should be over that by now.' He didn't actually say that, but that was his attitude. 'Well, do you want to go to Cruse?' [bereavement support group], and I thought, 'Well, I would like to go *on* a cruise,' but I said 'No, I have dealt with it for eight months, I think I can cope now.'
>
> (Janet)

Charmaz (1980) argues that the individualization of grief, which leaves people without social support, may be the very cause of the high disease and death rates identified in the newly bereaved. Her insight offers a key to understanding how the study of grief lost its way. It is not so much that the research findings are wrong at a descriptive level. It is true, for example, that people visit their doctor more frequently after a partner dies (Parkes 1964b) and that they are more likely to suffer a premature death than their non-bereaved contemporaries (Parkes *et al.* 1969), but that the very conception of the source of grief as an individual experience was wrong. To become bereaved we have to lose another person and it was the exclusion of the social and cultural aspect of loss that led grief studies down a blind alley. Thus, while the lists of psychological and physiological symptoms of normal bereavement such as restlessness, insomnia, weight-loss, feelings of anger and waves of hopelessness, etc. (Clayton *et al.* 1968; Faschingbauer *et al.* 1977; Parkes 1970, 1986; Raphael 1984; Zisook *et al.* 1982) meticulously collected from samples of predominantly white widows and widowers remain valid, it is just that this reductionist conceptualization of this experience does not really offer us great insights. I would argue that, as long as culture is reduced to a list of poorly defined variables and as long as the mind of the grieving individual is presumed to be asocial then we can hope for little understanding of the profound nature of loss.

Lay models of grief

Identifying phases and stages can act as a comforting displacement for those very people who are suffering from the sorrow of a bereavement. I found much evidence to support this. Indeed, the women often used medical metaphors to describe their grief, which was likened to surgery 'without anaesthetic' and of 'opening the wound'. Representations of the medical model of grief abound in our culture and it is not difficult to see how we access them. The representation of grief as disease has undergone subtle distortions during its passage from the 'scientific' world of psychiatry and psychology to the media world of soaps, documentaries, women's magazines and Sunday papers. Another source of norms of behaviour in grief come from the professionals, such as nurses, doctors and counsellors. Several of the women in my sample had received bereavement counselling. People also learned about their 'condition' from the community of other widows. One-third of people over 65 are bereaved (Bowling and Cartwright 1982). My respondents spent a great deal of time in the company of other women who had lost their husbands and listening to them talk about the advice they got from widowed friends. I sometimes felt they had almost undergone an apprenticeship. The women developed lay ideas concerning the grief reaction and were busy identifying stages and phases of their grief. The way in which this lay representation of grief has become distorted in its passage from person to person sometimes had serious repercussions. For example, Christine genuinely thought she would 'go through' all three stages.

I mean, a friend of mine told me there are three stages you go through when you lose someone. First of all you can't believe it, then you go through a stage of anger and then in the end you accept it. But, I certainly haven't got to anger yet.

(Christine)

I got upset . . . and you suffer all the things – well, now I hear that {'regrets'} is a stage we all go through.

(Paula)

The fear that grief can go wrong seems to run deep. Given a natural desire to present a 'healthy' model of grief to me, I sometimes had the feeling that the women thought there was some kind of hidden agenda to the interviews and that they did not want to sound as if they had 'unhealthy' grief reactions. You may remember that Susan telephoned to call me the day after the interview (see p. 160). On the other hand, they were highly motivated to make me aware of just how bad it was to lose a husband.

Everyone had absorbed the idea of 'grief work'. Some women discussed the need to 'talk out' and 'let out' dangerous build-ups of emotion. It was often hard for my respondents to find someone to listen to them, for the very person they usually confided in was gone. Susan turned to an old friend who lent an ear whenever she felt she had to talk. Other women felt it was more appropriate to hide signs of their grief as they believed that this was something they should not share with others. Paula congratulated herself on returning to work two days after her husband died. She felt this was a sign of a healthy ability to cope with her loss. When Kate's concerned daughters telephoned to see how she was doing she would often invent little white lies, such as a Sunday lunch date, in order to demonstrate that all was fine. Meanwhile, moments of complete despair, such as those described in some detail to me by Paula, were kept 'backstage'.

Even those who are sharing a loss can remain feeling alone. Isolated in two islands of sorrow Janet and her son, who lived with her, had hardly spoken to each other for months. Although Janet acknowledged that he was devastated by his dad's death, she was too intimidated by his coping façade to tackle the topic. She herself admitted that the exercise of self-control had became something of a source of satisfaction to her.

But, I, er, I think we are doing it for each other, to be quite honest. I won't break down, because of him, and he won't, for me

. . . He wouldn't even mention his father's name. He would walk out the door . . . [My husband] was television mad and football mad and [my son] is too, and I would say 'just like your father', and that. But he would walk out. I tried to bring him out but he [wouldn't] talk about him . . . He used to come in from work, go straight into [the] back room, where he always sat with his father. Because I was always in here, sort of doing things, he was always in there with his father.

(Janet)

This privatization of grief does not suit the women's purposes in the long run. It appears to create a feeling of generalized resentment towards others who, because they do not experience the pain of loss, are felt to underestimate it.

Yes. 'I am fine' . . . I make a joke, I am the same me. Totally independent, totally un-needy. And nobody knows basically, how I feel. Because I don't tell them. I don't show it.

(Paula)

I found that the saddest legacy of the medical model of grief was the widespread misconception of recovery. Some of my respondents were fighting with the contradictory experience of their feelings of desolation with the seemingly unattainable expectation of getting better, of being their old selves again. That their old self had 'died' along with their partners was not culturally accessible information; this seemed to make their sorrow even harder to bear.

I think my own expectation is as unreasonable as other people's in fact. One begins to think, 'Is it going to [go]?' And every time there is a good day I naïvely think, 'Oh good, I am better now.'

(Susan)

The resocialization of grief

My weekends are my worse point. It is very depressing, boring. The weekends. The week I find I can get through, sail through. But the weekends, I do get very strung up.

(Janet)

In qualitative studies we do not set the agenda in quite the same way that we do in quantitative research. As I mentioned in Chapter 2, the kind of information I got from the bereaved women who spoke to me was very different from what I had expected, given my background reading in the psychopathologies of grief. My interviewees often looked a little dishevelled and the stress and strain of the last few months was often made all too apparent by dark shadows under their eyes and their rather gaunt features. But rather than dwell on descriptions of symptoms of their grief they focused on their experience of loss. They told me about the death and their feelings about it. They described the ordeal of making funeral arrangements and talked about what it was like to be a single woman when all their friends seemed to still have living husbands. In this sense, getting information about the experience of grief was always by proxy. It was not at the forefront of the women's minds. This may sound as if this was an artefact of the research, simply a sign that I did not ask about their grief reaction. But I would argue that it was not that I did not ask, but that the experience of grief is always mediated by society and culture. It only gets separated and isolated when the research tools are specifically designed to remove those aspects of culture.

> What I needed at the time was practical help. And that I didn't get. It would have been marvellous if somebody had made me a soup . . . If somebody had come with a bowl of soup, [it would have been] a blessing. If somebody had come and wheeled my dustbin to where it should go . . . coming without asking, with something.
>
> (Ruth)

So the data which I worked on was a very different crop from the one I had expected to harvest. In a description of the experience of grief of elderly widows in which the researchers focused on their material circumstances, Bowling and Cartwright (1982) describe bereavements as a crisis in which the bereaved faced a range of problems 'from housing to health, loneliness to lethargy, and penury to the practicalities of day-to-day living' (1982: 1) (see also Marris 1958, 1986). Their research focused on the ways in which the bereaved are not just grieving but also finding themselves in a new state. My research findings seem to echo this.

> When a husband dies, you still got all them bills coming in . . . There is still the rent, the heating, everything, is exactly the same, but you are that man's money short.
>
> (Janet)

No description of bereavement would be complete without an emphasis on the huge practical strain put on people by the loss of a partner. For nearly all the women in my sample, finding enough money to run the household was a worry. With a traditional division of labour, many women were completely dependent on their husband's income. In these instances, the bereavement coincided with a new job for the widow. Even those who were relatively well off found dealing with their finances stressful. As Beth said, 'It would be useful to know how long you were going to live – then you could budget.'

The social nature of loss was articulated by the women when they came to give me advice to an imaginary newly bereaved person. This was one of the few questions I allowed myself to ask. It was posed at the end of the interview in order to lighten the atmosphere a little. This did not always work. The advice given is redolent with the isolation and loneliness felt by bereaved people nowadays. Warnings were given to the imaginary woman that other people will communicate poorly, avoid her when they can and, at times, behave badly towards her. Advice centred on her preparing to ride the waves upon waves of shock caused by losing a partner as she realizes, too late, that it was he who apparently earned all the money, ran the home, knew how to start the car, was the one people really liked, could talk to the teenage son and held the key to the very reason for her living.

> Do exactly what you want, not what others want. Because it will stay with you for a long, long time. Perhaps for ever.
>
> (Ruth)

Bereavement as a loss of self and other

> So I don't want to visit. Although I do, for company, but I feel that I am intruding. Because there should be two of me, but whereas two women can sit in the kitchen, have a jaw, while the two men will be in the front room watching football, it is not that now. So if I am in the kitchen with the wife, the husband is left on his own. You know, and you feel that you are taking something away, you know, from the man. It might not be right but that is the feeling you get.
>
> (Janet)

Mead (1934) argued that the mind is inherently social and depends on self–other relationships for its development. When the 'other' dies the social nature of the self becomes painfully obvious; for the very conception of self is threatened. Thus it is not only the loss of the 'other' but also the loss of 'self' that was partly constructed through interaction with the deceased other that makes grief the profound, painful and confusing experience it is. It is not just the sharing of public and private mourning practices that makes grief a social phenomenon.

In this conception of grief, what have been called the vulnerability factors – such as the class, sex or religiosity of the person suffering from the loss – are organically subsumed under the rubric of 'culture'. If we relinquish the erroneous belief that there are a set of natural laws to be discovered concerning the form and character of grief then culture is no longer reduced to a set of troublesome variables.

This notion of a socialized grief helps to explain cross-cultural differences. In line with Charmaz (1980) and Huntington and Metcalf (1979), I suggest that the *experience* of grief of other peoples is, at times, profoundly different precisely because these participants are adopting different sets of roles (Hochschild 1979; Averill 1982). That is not to say that the individuals who make up the group do not feel intense sorrow nor that in any way their expressions of grief are inauthentic or 'faked' (Hockey 1993). It is just that their experience of life and death is mediated through their cosmologies of the world and their belief systems concerning love, kinship, friendship, health and illness.

Reinstating culture to the scene also explains our own historical changes in the way we represent and experience grief (Ariès 1974; Dixon 1989; Jalland 1989; Laurence 1989).

> The psychologists have unwittingly made their analyses of mourning into an historical document, a proof of historical relativity. Their thesis is that the death of the loved one is a deep wound.
>
> (Ariès 1983: 581)

Once we have adopted such a position, certain characteristics of bereavement fall into place. First, the conception that we can recover or get better can be seen to be impossible. What is possible, however, is that the self should change. It is the rebuilding of the self that takes time, not the healing of an injury or wound. Such a view of bereavement has a lot in common with Kelly's (1955) personal construct theory, in which the grieving person is conceptualized as changing their personal construct systems, through the processes of dislocation and adaptation, in the face of the loss (see Raphael 1984: 69).

I knew when my husband died that the worst thing in life has happened to me. And in some ways that even was a comfort . . . Before it was my cancer, which preoccupied my thoughts sometimes.

(Ruth)

There are signs that conceptions of grief are changing. Significantly, many of the authors of recent volumes about loss are not psychologists. For example in *How We Grieve, Relearning the World*, Attig (1996) draws heavily on Heidegger (1962) in order to emphasize the importance of acknowledging the social nature of bereavement.

When someone in our world dies, we remain postured in that world as we were before the death, but we can no longer sustain that posture. We are challenged to learn new ways of feeling, behaving, thinking, expecting, and hoping in the aftermath of the loss. As we learn these things, we cope. Grieving, by definition, is just such coping with the challenges that bereavement presents. Grieving is what we do in response to what happens to us in bereavement.

(Attig 1996: viii)

In another recently published volume, Davies (1997) critiques the medical models of grief in which time is seen as a healer, an opportunity for the bereaved to return to normal. Focusing on rituals of bereavement, he argues that participation in funerals brings about changes in people. He describes funerals as our prime mode of defence. Having experienced such transcendence of ritual, bereaved people can themselves offer help to others who lose someone they love. These 'words against death' (1997: 1) have power because they are 'words invested with significance because of what they have experienced in the face of grief' (1997: 42).

Living with the dead

There is another characteristic of bereavement which could never really be satisfactorily explained within the medical model. This is the well-documented phenomenon of bereaved people maintaining the relationship with the dead via hallucinations, dreams and visions. Initially viewed as a manifestation of pathology, the presence of hallucinations was found to be so common that it had to be conceptualized as part of normal bereavement (Rees 1971; Yamamoto *et al.*

1969). Within the biology of grieving such findings never quite sat comfortably (see Ramsay 1977).

> No, I can't accept it. I mean, I know he has gone. But you know? But it's like, when I go out I still expect him to be there when I get back. I just can't . . .
>
> (Christine)

Klass (1995), in an analysis of parental bereavement, argues that parents in his study continued a relationship with an 'inner representation' of the dead child (Fairbairn 1952). Klass found that such representations lead to the sense of the deceased's presence, hallucinations, and the feeling that the child still has an active influence over events in the surviving parents' lives. The grieving parents also showed signs of having incorporated certain characteristics of their lost child into themselves. He argued that these manifestations were not simply individual phenomena but were 'maintained and reinforced within families and other social systems' (Klass 1995: 246). Based on research in contemporary America, his findings suggest that in this sense the dead child operates much as an ancestor, increasing the sense of closeness and interdependency between the surviving family members. Klass's (1995) descriptions of grieving, in which he explores the role of spirituality (seen as separate from religiosity, although often the two are linked) in loss, seem many light-years away from the modern, medical formulations of the grief reaction.

Obituaries in local newspapers are often full of these 'conversations with the dead'. As J. Davies (1996) notes, these informal, loving conversations are redolent with the ways in which the dead continue to occupy the world of the living. In my study I found expressions of this nature were very common, particularly when talking about making choices concerning the funeral. The lively way in which the women described their husbands' deathly wants were both touching and sad.

> It worried me that he was in a mortuary. I didn't want him in a mortuary, I wanted him to be in a private chapel of rest. I didn't want him there at all. And all I could keep seeing was these boxes, you know, knowing what they do. And I wanted him out of there.
>
> (Paula)

Several of the women I spoke to continued to have relationships with their dead husbands. Indeed, they found the possibility of communicating with them helpful in their period of intense loss. I was stuck by these on-going relationships with the husband after death. Based on years of habit, the women continued to imagine how their husbands would react to new situations. The bouncing of ideas of the phantasmal other could be remarkably effective. For, after decades of marriage, these women could imaginatively enter the dead man's mind in order to retrieve whatever advice or support they needed. This helped them. Paula, for example, believed that Reg watched her dress each morning. She would see him sitting up in bed, as he always used to. She chatted to him about the forthcoming day and would often consult him concerning what to wear. He would talk back to her: 'Your tag is sticking out' (dress label), he would say, or 'Oh, don't wear that!'

The women also held angry conversations with the deceased. They would complain about how hard life had become, moan about their lack of money or the complexity of probate and wish out loud that it was they who had died first. These arguments were seen to be particularly refreshing. However, the women's accounts of visions and visitations of the dead were not always comfortable ones and there was a certain amount of fear surrounding these sightings. Bloch and Parry (1982) note, despite the fact that the existence of ghosts is not acknowledged in the Bible, that the Christian world has always feared such hauntings from the dead (see Hallam *et al.* forthcoming).

Forget-me-not

I have got him in the 'book of remembrance', up at the crematorium. I have got a miniature iris at the side, they have done it beautifully, they do them beautifully, you know, and I have found a verse.

(Paula)

The strength of this relationship gives us an insight into the motivations behind the widespread and popular practice of memorialization (Bradbury 1993b). The fact that people spend so much time choosing and visiting memorials makes a lot more sense when we appreciate the vibrancy of the post-mortem relationship. Memorialization is not something that is particularly positively sanctioned at the moment. It is often seen as an expression of a psychopathology, a failure to let go and move on. Our ambivalent feelings about the concrete expression of loss through the purchase of memorials may reflect our sense of unease about the survivors sustaining a relationship with people who are dead.

Yet people often spend a great deal of money on memorials, which is always an indication that something is important to us in this culture. I found that my respondents were often slightly sheepish about their purchases, admitting to the considerable sums spent on rose bushes and entries in books of remembrance with some reluctance. Some are not permitted the luxury of feeling guilty. Christine was very distressed that she had not been able to afford an entry in the book of remembrance. Adrift in grief she bemoaned the fact that there was no memorial to her husband. For those who did have the money, the visits to their memorial site afforded them an opportunity to carry out their conversations with the deceased. Most people developed a pattern of visiting structured around personal anniversaries and public holidays. They engaged in a variety of activities while there. They cleaned, gardened and adorned their memorials, often engaging in conversation with their husbands while they did their memorial housework. This touching care of the memorial seemed a natural extension of their conjugal relationship (see Bradbury forthcoming).

> I like to go. I take up my little gloves, and my bits, you know. And just walk over there and make sure it is all tidy, make sure that the roses are okay.
>
> (Janet)

Summary and conclusion

> I think I am beginning to understand why grief feels like suspense. It comes from the frustration of so many impulses that had become habitual. Thought after thought, feeling after feeling, action after action, had H. for their object. Now their target has gone. I keep on through habit fitting an arrow to the string; then I remember and have to lay the bow down.
>
> (Lewis 1961: 41)

In this chapter I have been looking at our social representations of grief and bereavement. The universal experience of loss has been objectified in the modern era. Described in terms of disease with an easy-to-recognize symptomatology, health-care professionals were quick to adopt this model. Indeed the search for desirable and undesirable outcomes and the goal of recovery was quickly disseminated to the lay population. As the field of study enlarged, new models of grief were developed, such as the stage–phase models inspired by the hospice movement. While attempting to develop a more humane view on loss, the stage–phase model of grief continued to be dogged by the implicit assumption that there were good or bad ways of grieving. These models have proved to be enduringly popular.

I have been arguing that the quest to understand why people had different grief outcomes illuminated a flaw in this individualized model of grief. Those 'risk factors' which were envisioned to cluster around an isolated and vulnerable person would be better viewed as the culture in which people live. The conceptualization of grief as a disease was doomed to failure because it did not take into account the role played by changing representations of death in Britain's recent social history. For example, there are significant generational differences in the ways in which people express their emotions. These differences are not just shaped by questions of age, but by social norms which go in and out of fashion. An appreciation of the cultural relativity of emotion also helps to explain the subtle cross-cultural differences in the expression and experience of loss and grief.

Thus, models of grief reflect our current social representations of life and death and for this reason they can date fast. I have not attempted to construct yet another model of grief, but I have merely offered an alternative perspective on an experience that is a normal part of our lives. The concept of loss needs to be resocialized. I have argued that grief is a social phenomenon, dependent on other people. When someone we love dies it is not just the loss of the other that gives rise to the psychological and physiological distress that has been meticulously noted by psychiatrists and psychologists over the last 50 years, but the loss of self. Rebuilding a new self takes time as the loss of the beloved 'other-half' is incorporated into this new, post-bereavement self. Thus a part of this self includes a space for a continuing relationship with the dead person. As Attig (1996) puts it 'making the transition from loving persons who are present to loving them in their absence' (1996: ix).

8 Re-presenting death

Without realizing it, I entered the field during a quiet revolution in contemporary deathways. Most of my research findings slotted into that now-familiar duo of the sequestration and privatization of death. Other data, however, did not fit this formulation. I was coming across self-reflexive respondents (see Giddens 1991), who had become active agents for the dying, death and disposal of their next of kin. While remaining customers, these people were anything but passive 'clients'. In this final chapter I draw my research findings together within a framework of sociological social psychology. The first section focuses on the work of Goffman before ending with a discussion of the relevance of Mead's philosophy of the self and Moscovici's theory of social representations.

The social organization of death

As other authors have observed (Prior 1989), there is no doubt that the social organization of death is dominated by bureaucracy and medical science. Even the calmest and most expected death involves at least five institutions and is likely to lead to the employment of six or seven different kinds of deathworker. More complicated deaths – those which happen unexpectedly or in suspicious circumstances – will cause the employment of yet more deathworkers and other types of professionals, such as the police or barristers. Moving along from institution to institution, from one deathworker to another, there are few constants in the social organization of death. The corpse and the next of kin are the two main participants; they are the only 'actors' to partipate in the whole play through its various stages.

As Goffman notes (1961: 290) over the last 100 years there has been a tendency for the 'tinkering services' to move away from pedlars' carts and home visits to the 'workshop complex', in which the potential customer becomes the consumer. This is very much the case with the social organization of death. The 'clients' visit the 'server' in a series of 'workshops': the hospital mortuary, the funeral parlour and the crematorium. These are designed and built for the purpose and aid the policing of both the public and the private spaces. At each site are placed professionals who have been trained in certain specialized roles and who take over at the required moment. These deathworkers deal with death on a daily basis; they compartmentalize and professionalize their strange tasks and jobs. Many of them are in a 'personal-service occupation': that is, they perform a 'specialised personal service' for a set of individuals involving personal communication (Goffman 1961: 284). In return, each client brings respect, trust, gratitude and a fee.

In a society that tends to give 'professionals' extraordinary freedoms and status, it is not surprising to find that deathworkers resort to a strategy of 'professionalizing' their jobs. Yet the physical nature of death does not always lend itself to the kind of order and decorum 'professionalism' would imply. So our death practices are permeated by a certain detectable tension. Many deathworkers do not really qualify for professional status at all, but we have to remember that they do have special skills. We no longer know how to lay-out a body for example. This particular art has been lost for at least a generation. The professional practitioner's job is made all the stranger by the confusion over who, precisely, the client is: is it the corpse or the next of kin? While the corpse does not purchase memorial stones, earlier in its voyage through the social organization of death it was a living patient, indisputably the client. This shifting role between client and object can create unusual situations. For example, on occasion, a dying person may wish to have an interview with the funeral director to arrange their own funeral.

The corpse as an object presents an unusual problem. Unlike the majority of objects in our world, ownership is ambiguous. As a possession, it has a status not dissimilar to that of bodily waste, such as faeces or blood. Yet just as blood used for transfusion can be seen to be 'valuable', the corpse has moments of symbolic, legal and monetary value. Officially, the corpse is the legal possession of the next of kin, unless the cause of the death is in dispute, in which case the Crown, i.e. government, assumes ownership. In reality the police, coroner and pathologist take over this investigatory role. Thus the bereaved 'client's' ownership of the object may be tenuous. Informally, for example, a doctor or consultant may feel it to be within their moral rights to put pressure on the next of kin to get permission for a post-mortem for the purposes of research.

The deathwork professional has gained control of our dead. The professionals' possession of the symbolically and commercially powerful corpse puts this beyond dispute. Possession is the key to power. Throughout the first week of mind-numbing bureaucracy great care is taken to ensure that whichever professional is in 'play' at any particular moment has the body: either physically, such as the funeral director's keeping the body in his parlour, or bureaucratically, such as the coroner's 'holding' the body in the hospital mortuary. This overrides genuine questions of ownership and we are generally left in ignorance as to our precise rights concerning the corpse. Few relatives ever know that it is possible to keep the body at home in the week before disposal or that, having received permission, they may bury the dead outside a church or cemetery wall.

A dramaturgical approach

> A correctly staged and performed scene leads the audience to impute a self to a performed character, but this imputation – this self – is a *product* of a scene that comes off, and is not a *cause* of it. The self, then as a performed character, is not an organic thing that has a specific location, whose fundamental fate is to be born, to mature, and to die; it is a dramatic effect arising diffusely from a scene that is present, and the characteristic issue, the crucial concern, is whether it will be credited or discredited.
>
> (Goffman 1959: 245)

Goffman (1959) argued that the very structure of the self can be seen in terms of how we make presentations of ourselves to others. In the first week following a death bereaved people are thrown into a series of exchanges with deathwork professionals. Both sets of people attempt to maintain an orderly presentation of self under what are extraordinary circumstances.

In any social situation the individual, in this case the bereaved client, wishes to perceive events realistically. Yet as Goffman (1959) notes, information is rarely complete so the individual has to rely on cues, hints, expressive gestures, status symbols, etc. In short they have to go on appearances. Goffman claims that the impressions given off by others are treated as promises or claims that, morally, should be fulfilled. Meanwhile the perceived, such as the deathworker, are expected to act as if they were unaware that impressions about them are being formed. But at times it is necessary for the deathworker to manipulate the impressions they give off. As Goffman (1959) puts it 'the observed become a performing team and the observers become the audience. Actions which appear to be done on objects become gestures addressed to the audience. The round of activity becomes dramatised' (Goffman 1959: 243).

When someone dies, impression management is put under a certain strain. Usually in work situations each actor attempts to achieve a reasonably coherent performance. This performance relies on the management of expressive acts and on the use of props. In death, all too easily, impression management, on both the part of the professional and the bereaved, can come unstuck. The funeral directors are acutely aware of this and their talk is scattered with anecdotes of disasters, when their 'front' was torn down. This sharing of anecdotes undoubtedly plays an important role in maintaining their determination to isolate the public from things that will disturb them and, thereby, threaten the professionals' carefully contrived social construction of death.

A grieving person, most of the time, is as concerned about impression management as everyone else. Their efforts to maintain a stiff upper lip, or to appear to display appropriate grief (i.e. as medically healthy or fit) can also lead them, like the deathwork professional, to create a dramatic world. The team is made up of family and friends and the 'props' include letters of condolence, flowers, candles, even old answerphone cassettes that hold a recording of that much missed and dearly loved voice. Backstage, there may be moments in which the real character of loss is expressed in terms of outbursts or quiet moments of reflection in which communication with the deceased takes the form of conversations, prayers, hallucinations and dreams. Too soon the survivors have to gather their resources for yet another performance.

Being a deathworker is very stressful. The timing and manner of death can be unpredictable, the corpse can be repulsive and the bereaved are distraught and liable to outbursts of one kind or another. Goffman (1961: 78) notes that 'people work' differs from other kinds of work because of the 'tangle of statuses and relationships' that characterize it. Actions surrounding the corpse and its next of kin are heavily influenced by the human nature of the object. When things do go wrong the results are disastrous. Such is the deathworker's desire to deal with each death smoothly and efficiently that their clients are not told about mistakes, hitches and hold-ups. People should, ideally, politely ignore any gaffs, but there is no guarantee that a grief-stricken person will calmly or tactfully turn a blind eye. Emotions are running too high. So when Christine saw the funeral director's men bundling her husband's body into a body bag she did not simply turn away as she was supposed to. Instead she ran into the room, screaming and weeping, and tore at the zip they were trying to close (see p. 77).

> Within the walls of a social establishment we find a team of performers who cooperate to present to an audience a given definition of the situation. This will include the conception of own team and of audience and assumptions concerning the ethos that is to be maintained by rules of politeness and decorum. We often find a division into back region, where the performance of a routine is prepared, and front region, where the performance is presented. Access to these regions is controlled to prevent the audience from seeing backstage and to prevent outsiders from coming into a performance that is not addressed to them.
>
> (Goffman 1961: 231)

The manner in which deathworkers work as a loosely knit team will have already become apparent. As I mentioned, a great deal of energy goes into presenting a smooth front to the bereaved client. Within the trade those deathworkers who have a clash of interests and who, backstage, can be quite antagonistic, assume a friendly demeanour towards each other the moment a member of the public is close by. Thus the mild state of war that exists between certain clergy and funeral directors continues unnoticed by the thousands of people who employ them.

Keeping the show on the road may involve telling white lies. Thus a dismembered arm is carefully sutured back on in the embalming room and no one is the wiser (see p. 127). Maintaining this front certainly requires a degree of privacy. The various sites or workshops in which the professionals deal with the dying and the dead are carefully split into front and back stages. This use of front and backstage areas to aid the practice of staff was also demonstrated by Glaser and Strauss (1965, 1968) in their seminal work on dying in hospitals. The grieving family are excluded from those areas in which the body is manhandled or, most importantly, changed. The most traumatic acts – post-mortem, refrigeration, embalming, dressing and finally cremation – take place out of view. Most of these acts, except for dressing, are reasonably recent developments. Burial, in contrast, still takes place frontstage. This is a reflection of the increasing distance placed between the mourners and the corpse.

However, people inevitably get the occasional, sneaked glimpse behind the scenes. These are vividly remembered. Even when they are successfully excluded, they use their imaginations to colour-in the sections of the social organization of death hidden from their view. With the acute concentration that loss brings, people create a strange world of death practices in which they draw on both ancient and modern images of death. Precisely because they are uncertain what the mortuary looks like they imagine overflowing mortuaries with refrigerated cubicles, drawers agape. Precisely because they do not know what is behind the crematorium curtain through which the coffin slides, they picture blazing furnaces, 'live cremations' and an obscene mixing of the resulting ashes.

Excluding the bereaved family and friends from the backstage areas in which the body is held, disempowers them. On the one hand the deathwork professional, in their efforts to keep control of the corpse and what happens to it, is sometimes viewed with ill-disguised distrust. On the other hand, it is precisely the ignorance of what happens backstage that facilitates the mythification of the deathwork professional. The doctor becomes God and (as one woman put it) the funeral director the 'knight in shining armour'. This tendency to idealize is very human. In such a time of confusion and chaos, it is reassuring to believe in someone.

So our experience of the death of a significant other is thus artificially fed to us through a series of 'frontstage' areas. To a certain extent, the first week following the death can be characterized as a series of queues in private waiting-rooms and a series of interviews with professionals and pseudo-professionals in pseudo-office spaces together with endless cups of tea or coffee. Current grief therapies, developed to help us, invariably involve even more talk. If a death is in any way spectacular, grieving relatives may also expect to attract the interest of the mass media, keen for personal accounts from family members.

Interspersed with this waiting and being interviewed are moments of pure drama in which the professionals present and represent the ever-changing corpse. Disinherited from the age-old rights of intimacy (washing and dressing the body, etc.) and control over the corpse, the bereaved family and friends can only hope to meet the body at these specific points in its passage from the newly dead to either ashes or soil. These potentially explosive meeting points take place in frontstage areas that are carefully controlled—staged by the professionals. At these moments props such as flowers, dress, lighting and hymns are used.

Goffman (1959) argued that his theatrical metaphor should be viewed as simply a metaphor. He emphasized that while a theatrical show was only a presentation of a reality, life is a reality, with real consequences. The split between what is real and what is theatre is particularly hazy in the social organization of death, as certain aspects of this organization are highly ritualistic in character. As a sociologist, interested in institutions, Goffman presumably did not have rituals and customs in mind. The sense of unrealness, or pure theatre, in our death rituals should not be underestimated. I argue that despite the ways in which death has become controlled by medical science and appropriated by commerce, contemporary British funerals can still operate as rituals in which the participants undergo a transformation.

Socializing death

In the previous chapter I explored how a Meadian view of mind, self and society might enable us to grasp the meaning of loss and bereavement in new terms. Central to my thesis regarding the social construction of death has been the argument that mind is socially constructed.

> We must regard mind, then, as arising and developing within the social process, within the empirical matrix of social interactions. We must, that is, get an inner individual experience from the standpoint of social acts which include the experiences of separate individuals in a social context wherein those individuals interact.
>
> (Mead 1934: 133)

Mind is thus created when, in social interaction, the individual becomes self-conscious and, in turn, relegates their experience to memory. Mead suggests that the 'self' arises in the process of social experience and activity. Adopting such a position helps us to understand how we represent death. If mind itself is socially constructed then clearly the ways in which we represent death also exist as a result of social exchange. These socially constructed representations in turn shape our current death practices.

When someone we love dies we are plunged into an unusual, threatening and distressing set of circumstances where nothing is as it was. We find ourselves taking part in a series of elaborate cultural acts and complex discourses which, for many of us, miraculously give some sense of meaning to the death, despite all the pain of loss and grief that accompanies that understanding. In Chapter 1 I argued that it should be possible to develop a social psychological perspective on death and dying. In this section I return to the theory of social representations.

Customs, rituals and representations

It is commonly accepted that contemporary death practices are perfunctory, empty and without old-style customary and ritual power. I disagree. It is simply that we fail to see where our customs and death rituals are flourishing. It appears that we are blind to our own cultural ingenuity, while remaining locked into a collective nostalgia.

The following acts are significant social customs in contemporary London: certifying and registering the cause of death, the viewing and embalming of the corpse, placing notices in papers, the funeral cortège, the cremation ceremony (when non-religious), the use of cards and letters of condolence and the sending of flowers. The following would appear to fit the description of ritual acts, although what makes a ritual authentic relies on the meaning extracted by the participants, not on the objects which are used as props: the funeral service, certain burial and cremation rites, some wakes and memorial services and personal rites centring on memorial objects. For many people in Britain today, death rituals do have an existential dimension. Indeed, for a lucky few the participation in ritual can afford the opportunity to transcend death altogether. The structure and lay-out of the funeral parlour and the crematorium, the black hearse, the show-room full of coffins and the touching epithets to be found in the book of remembrance all could be viewed as objectifications, expressed as part of the ritual process, of our representations of death as rebirth. However, as Moscovici (1984a) most certainly did not have custom and ritual in mind when he described the processes of objectification and anchoring it is possible that another process is at work, such as symbolization. Indeed, Joffe (1999) has noted that there is a great deal of overlap between objectification and symbolization.

Douglas (1966) states that, the modern Western world does not utilize or display neat patterns of pollution fears as the fabric of our society is too complex. However, it is possible to identify strange systems of belief that cluster around areas of ambiguity. These unfamiliar terrains are a source of ritual power. We have some less-than-fully rational feelings about the dead body, which is subject to strong pollution taboos. Precisely because of its decomposing and inert condition it is a singularly rich source for symbols. The things that we do to the body, such as dressing it, embalming it, encoffining it, viewing it, cremating and/or burying it cannot be explained in purely rationalist terms. Harnessing our fears of pollution we make the corpse express our representations of life and death.

So, contemporary mortuary practices cannot be dismissed as some kind of ritual shadows. We all face questions of mortality, whatever our culture. British representations of death are not only to be found in medical practice (science) or films, documentaries and newspapers (media), they also exist in our death customs and rituals. These customary and ritual acts are replete with meaning. They express our representations of death, serving as both vehicles of traditional representations and the means of effecting change. Like those of other cultures, the customs and rituals of our society are almost invisible and, for many, taking part in them can be a comfortable, almost mundane, experience.

> The purpose of all representations is to make something unfamiliar, or unfamiliarity itself, familiar.
>
> (Moscovici 1984a: 25)

The study of death would appear to provide an excellent opportunity for observing the processes whereby people make the unfamiliar familiar. What is unfamiliar about death is relatively obvious: the inert state of the body of a relative or patient; the body's remorseless change from human corpse to rotting carcass; the strange and unpredictable behaviour of the grieving relative; the loss of family or friend or work roles. The list goes on. Almost everything about death seems unfamiliar. Probably this is true for all cultures. However, in the industrialized West, unfamiliarity is increased by two further factors. First, as I mentioned in Chapter 6, large numbers of the urban population are alienated from the natural world and do not often, if ever, see dying or dead animals. Second, the social organization of death is in the hands of a small group of professionals who guard their activities as jealously as the members of a medieval guild ever did.

> The representations we fabricate – of a scientific theory, a nation, an artefact, etc. – are always the result of a constant effort to make usual and actual something which is unfamiliar or which gives us a feeling of unfamiliarity. And through them we overcome it and integrate it into our mental and physical world which is thus enriched and transformed.
>
> (Moscovici 1984a: 27)

Moscovici also considered those things that are 'like us, and yet not like us', such as the mentally ill and those from another culture. Moscovici suggested that those things that fail to become familiar are pushed aside and are likely to be endowed with imaginary, often negative, characteristics. This is typical of the 'unfamiliar'. Thus, the corpse and those who deal with it are marginalized and subject to negative and quite erroneous characterizations. Both the deathwork professionals and the next of kin are contaminated by their contact with the polluting corpse.

Moscovici (1984a) dismissed three other 'traditional' explanations of why we create representations, one of which is that groups create representations to filter information from the environment and thus control individual behaviour. While he acknowledges that there may be a certain amount of truth in this, his dismissal of this extremely significant explanation may have been over-hasty. After all, it would appear to be one of the implicit working hypotheses of many anthropological texts. For example, Bloch and Parry (1982) argue that the ritual celebration of death may be used to further those in power. This is doing more than just make the unfamiliar familiar. This theme of control can be seen to operate in modern society too. It is possible, for example, that the representation of the good medical death as painless was first created by doctors involved in a power struggle with the clergy at death beds during the nineteenth century. Medical practitioners continue to be involved in the promotion of the good medical death. This is to do with control, rather than with familiarization.

Re-presenting the good death

As we would expect, the dominant system into which the unfamiliar corpse and the recently bereaved are both integrated is that of the medical model. The unfamiliar corpse is anchored in medical knowledge. The dead body is treated much like a patient, the bereaved like the mentally ill. The classification and naming which is a sign that anchoring has taken place is centred on medical descriptions of the cause of death. This in turn feeds into a discourse about whether the death was good or bad.

There are other systems of classification. We also make use of age-old concepts of the sacred good death and the rebirth of the dying. When Moscovici first formulated the processes of anchoring and objectification he still had in mind the split between the reified world of science and the consensual world of common sense. Objectification, in particular, was envisaged as the process whereby intellectual ideas are made more concrete and physically accessible. Fortunately, the process of objectification still seems to make sense if we consensualize science. Once we have anchored a death into the context of medical science then we can objectify the death by delaying decomposition. To give another example: if we wish to construct the image of the medically controlled death it is possible to make this a physical reality by the application of fatal doses of opiates. Thus embalming and euthanasia become objectifications of our representations of the medical good death. Moscovici noted how we also objectify by means of language. The use of euphemisms and various labels peculiar to the funeral trade appear to fit this description. Embalming, for example, becomes 'hygienic treatment'.

While I set out to discover our current social representations of death, at the outset I was not sure what form these representations would assume. However, the anthropological and historical literature had provided me with some ideas, namely, that societies tend to shape deaths into those that are good, bad, natural and unnatural. It appears that Bloch and Parry's (1982) prediction that ideas of regeneration and rebirth are more weakly stressed in an industrialized, individualistic society is correct. However, we still need to anchor unfamiliar death and in this book I have tried to show how age-old representations of the good, bad, natural and unnatural death continue to be utilized by professionals and bereaved alike.

During the eighteenth and nineteenth century representations of dying changed along with medical innovations. Dying was increasingly viewed as a process that could be made painless through the application of powerful painkillers. With the development of a secular climate of opinion, however, not only did the manner of the good death change but also its meaning. In brief, for many people it became profane. The good death was no longer concerned with the fate of the soul; it was concerned only with the character of the physical event. The medical notion of good death continues to be the dominant representation of good deaths and the hospital environment appears to provide the optimal degree of control. We can manipulate the time, location and expression of death. So, with the exception of self-sacrifice or murder, medical science provides the best conditions for the human control and manipulation of the process of dying. Bloch and Parry (1982) suggest that the key to a good death is a sense of control. As it happens, the illusion of human control over life and death can be enjoyed from within the medical model and deaths that require some kind of medical intervention and/or hospitalization seem good candidates for becoming good deaths, as I found to be the case. The cause of death is of crucial importance to any type of good death because the type of disease has an impact on such factors as awareness, preparation and consciousness of the dying person.

Managing to orchestrate a medical good death has become the

concern of medical practitioners. However, as I mentioned earlier, this does not just influence the behaviour of medical personnel in the hospital, home or hospice. It has also influenced the behaviour of those deathwork professionals who deal with the corpse. The coroner, registrar and funeral director are all involved in a medical discourse about death that is partly concerned with presenting the image of the painless, sleep-like death. Deaths that do not conform to this stereotype – the bad medical deaths and particularly those that do not produce a reposeful corpse (Prior 1989: 160) – galvanize the deathwork professional into hiding or disguising the facts of the death (Bradbury 1996). This professional good practice is justified as being a way of protecting the bereaved. The professional's image of the bereaved, whose grief is potentially 'pathological', is engendered by the application of a medical model to grief as well as to the medical good and bad deaths.

In a reaction against a perceived excess of medical intervention in the process of dying, the term 'natural death' has recently enjoyed a comeback. While coroners' courts have been using the expression for some time, talk about dying 'naturally' was unfashionable during the modern era. With increasing longevity and changing death trajectories our conceptions of a good way of dying are being revolutionized. Rejecting scenarios that seem depersonalizing and over-medicalized, people are now exploring 'new' ways of dying. From the start the natural death movement cannily anchored itself in people's consciousness by affiliating itself with a very successful representation (and movement): the natural birth movement. There are many differences between giving birth and dying and the affinity between the two does not stand close scrutiny. Yet the use of the title worked and everyone, particularly the media, knew exactly what the movement's leaders were saying.

Moscovici described two roles of representations. The first is that they 'conventualise the objects, persons and events we encounter' (1984a: 7). The grouping of these objects, persons and events into models helps to structure an otherwise chaotic universe. So death is conventualized by the representations we have formed about the dead body and the grieving relative. The second is that they are prescriptive, 'that is, they impose themselves upon us with an irresistible force' (1984a: 9). Examples of the prescriptive nature of our representations of death abound. In our moment of deepest grief we warmly thank the doctor and are meticulously careful to be compliant, polite and composed. We find ourselves describing the deaths of our loved ones as good, although we are hard put to find a reason. Thus calling a death good or bad may not be about believing it is either good or bad, but simply gives the survivors a socially acceptable handle on this most taboo of topics. As Moscovici notes:

> By setting a conventional sign of reality on the one hand, and, on the other, by prescribing through tradition and age-old structures, *what* we perceive and imagine, these creatures of thought, which are representations, end up by constituting an actual environment.
>
> (Moscovici 1984a: 12, original italics)

Thus the anchoring of death as good or bad in sacred, medical or natural terms confines the participants to a pattern of behaviour and rules. Clearly the representation of the good or bad death is the concern of the living, yet it constrains those same people when it is their turn to die. I do not wish to suggest that this representation of death is used cynically by the professionals. They genuinely believe they are making life easier for the bereaved. Discussions by death-workers of their own experiences of bereavement suggest that they use the same representations of the good death when they lose someone they love. Significantly, I found that they appear just as vulnerable to conflict with those in control as the non-professional bereaved.

We do not just occupy roles like a theatre troupe (Goffman 1959). We also compete and argue. I agree with Billig (1986) in his call for the merging of the theatre and game metaphors. As I hope will have become apparent in Chapter 6, the discourse about the good and bad death is 'argumentative'. As Moscovici (1984a) notes, when one person's classification of an object or an event is imposed on another's they convey a bundle of expectations as to how the other person should respond. There is no guarantee that the other person will agree. I found that the bereaved kin were not at all passive about classifying their partner's death as good or bad and they certainly do not always share the same representation as the deathwork professional. We can observe a tussle for power in those instances where the bereaved's representations of death are not in accordance with those of the professionals'. We might imagine that the outcome of such negotiations or arguments would be predictable, given that the professional is usually in a position of power over their bereaved client. Yet I found that despite their distress, families stubbornly resist the constraints imposed by the professionals and the professionals' personal representation of the death, and still manage to win the day by reinstating their own personal representations after the disposal of the body.

We should be wary of constructing 'definitions' of the good death. Given the popularity of the good death in literature of the social sciences (Ariès 1974, 1983; Beier 1989; Bradbury 1993a, 1996; Kellehear 1990; Samerel 1995; Small 1993; Walter 1994) it is possible that the lay population will appropriate, and in the process distort, this 'scientific knowledge' about the good and bad ways of doing a death.

Re-presenting the healthy grief

Just as the medical model dominates our representations of the good and bad death, I have argued that grief has been similarly medicalized. For decades psychologists have viewed grief as the archetypal individual experience. Counsellors, therapists, journalists and the bereaved themselves have been looking for symptoms, stages and outcomes which they believe to be concrete phenomena, like a tumour or a fracture, rather than a social representation of loss. The anchoring of bereavement in the grief reaction simultaneously constrains the sorrowful person and reassures the observer about all those chaotic and powerful expressions of loss. That which was disturbing and unknown becomes the known, belonging to a category and with a familiar set of characteristics.

The psychiatric and psychological research into grief has failed to appreciate the social nature of grief as mourning individuals battle to rebuild their damaged selves. I found that my respondents had a notion of grief as something that might turn into a life-threatening disease. These women did not have to be apprenticed into knowing about this representation, for it permeates our popular culture. So just as I tapped into the representations of good and bad deaths as salient features in the interviews themselves, the psychiatric and psychological research into the grief reaction, discussed in the last chapter, tapped not the reality of grief as a disease but social representations of grief as a disease. Representations, however, have a habit of becoming realities. These studies remain fascinating and important, even though the psychiatrists and psychologists conducting them did not discover what they thought they had. The use of quantitative research tools, in which the researcher sets the agenda, may have obscured the process of re-presentation.

In conclusion

It has been argued that the postmodern era, which has been developing at some pace over the last few decades, represents a chance for the re-enchantment of society, a welcome return of the 'subject' (Bauman 1992b). However, there are problems associated with this. As Bauman notes 'the post-modern mind seems to condemn everything, propose nothing' (1992b: 9). The wholescale demolition and deconstruction of our modern and objective view of the world can engender fear of the void. Thus we attack the medical model and dismantle the safe, reassuring descriptions of the stages of dying, the good medical death and healthy grief and in their place seem to leave nothing but variety and choice. Incoherence seems to be postmodernism's distinctive feature. Bauman would argue that we are tearing down the power-supported structure of the modern era, the false truths that were constructed out of a desperate search for structure and order that followed on the heels of the Renaissance. But this does not lessen those private fears which are expressed in the contemporary mania for the DIY solutions poignantly illustrated by the natural death movement, in which dying individuals are encouraged to 'take on' their own deaths and to draw comfort from the imagined community of fellow natural death supporters.

Death is a physical event that turns the subjective self into an objective other and for this reason represents something of a challenge to our conception of this brave new world. My exploration of contemporary deathways revealed them to be both traditional and innovative. With apparent ease we seem to be able to accept both continuity and change, that fine balance which enables us to draw an embalmed corpse on a horse-drawn hearse to the local crematorium for a service with a priest.

Despite the rapid rate of change over the past couple of centuries there seems little sign that our belief in immortality has been genuinely deconstructed, thus causing an over-emphasis of the here and now which is so often described as a sign of postmodernism's hold over us (Bauman 1992b). There is little that is either 'ephemeral' or 'evanescent' about planting a tree or erecting a headstone (Bauman 1992b). Many of the social representations of death and the customs and rituals which express them do act as a balm to the survivors. These funerals are rites of passage which send our loved ones to the other world. There is symbolism to gather by the armful if we only know where to look: the floral tribute that shouts 'FOREVER'; the kitsch condolence card bedecked with doves; the visit to the funeral director's chapel to see a corpse pumped full of formaldehyde; the poem recited on a favourite hilltop as the wind catches the ashes as they are poured from their urn; the dedicated bench in the park. The British way of death cannot be explained away in terms of mindless tradition, the dominance of the medical profession or the seductive force of consumerism. These acts are full of the meanings of love, life and the hereafter.

Appendix

The analysis of data

Although the analysis of data went hand-in-hand with the data-collection process, it is useful to indicate how the data was analysed in a separate section. In this short appendix I discuss the analysis of the participant observation study and the in-depth interviews with twelve grieving women.

Analysing the participant-observation study

The first stage in the analysis of the data from the participant-observation study entailed a description of the characteristics of the community. Drawing on the fieldwork I began to plot out the general social organization of death. Listing the various deathwork professionals involved, I drew arrows between those who had contact with other professionals. I also made note of hierarchies and of who was obliged to contact who. For example, funeral directors are supposed to inform the local clergy that a death has taken place in their parish, yet I found that many funeral directors do not do so. Perhaps surprisingly, many funeral directors perceive their status to be higher than that of the clergy. I discuss this in Chapter 4. Prior (1989: 29), drawing on the Consumers' Association guide *What to Do when Someone Dies* (Rudinger 1986), has already provided an excellent flow-chart that illustrates what happens after someone dies. I observed the actions and inter-actions between the deathwork professional, the corpse and the bereaved next of kin and developed my own chart. I wished to discern who, at any point in time, played a central or important role and who, if anyone or thing, was marginalized. I also adopted a chronological perspective from the moment of death, and logged the various phases through which the body and the bereaved relative pass: namely, the medical, bureaucratic, commercial and ritual domains, to reveal the last movements of the corpse before it came to its final resting place.

Turning to the transcripts of the key informants I then began my coding. I used the qualitative data analysis package 'Text-base Alpha'. This software allows you to code and sort long transcripts. You can scan down the text with the cursor and mark chunks of speech with various code names. You can apply multiple codes to the same phrase, sentence, paragraph or page. For example, Sharon, a nurse, made the following comment about death on the ward: 'We tend to walk out with them anyway. You tend to think that it is still a patient until you go out the door.' By which she meant that she accompanied the corpse to the exit of the ward, just as she would a live patient. I could code this text under 'deceased' (the codeword for examples in which professionals discussed their relationship with the deceased) and under 'body' (the code used whenever subjects discussed the corpse). During my analysis I could therefore use the same sentence to examine different shades of meaning. I could examine huge lists of decontextualized statements, made by different deathwork professionals, about the same topic, such as their view of the corpse or their relationship with the deceased. What was useful about these vast lists of decontextualized quotations was that it gave me the opportunity of rapidly comparing sets of comments and statements. The computer does the kind of sorting and organizing qualitative researchers used to do in their heads or with bits of coloured card. The quotations were never genuinely 'decontextualized' as I was the data-collector, transcriber and coder as well as the person who analysed them. Despite my familiarity with the data, I found that decontextualizing the text momentarily made the speech strange to me. It gave me the opportunity to see what was said with fresh eyes and at times shook my assumption that I understood what they were saying to me. Seconds later I would recognize the quotations and recontextualize them. But I could now understand them in a new light.

This computer package is dependent on a well-thought-out coding frame and it took several months to develop the coding frames to my satisfaction. My coding frame for the participant-observation key-informant interviews comprised more than 70 coding titles, such as 'awareness states' (code for comments by widow regarding her awareness of husband's impending demise); 'organ-harvesting' (code for accounts by professionals or bereaved relatives regarding requests for organs for donation) and 'cremate' (code for descriptions or comments regarding cremation). This coding frame could be broadly split into groups or clusters of codes which dealt with the following: the moment of death, aspects of medical intervention, descriptions of bureaucracy, statements about the bereaved client, discussions about the corpse, ritual aspects, relationships with other professionals, the label applied to a death (good, bad, natural) and to the dead (relative social value of different people, etc.), being a deathwork professional and the interview situation. In this final category I marked and coded those parts of an interview that were interrupted, or in which it appeared that the interviewee was uncomfortable, defensive, aggressive or just plain confused by my questioning.

Those who are being studied are, themselves, analytic. We can learn much from their ordering of events and ideas. An example of a 'participant' concept, or code, is the 'good death', which is part of the jargon used by both the deathwork professional and the bereaved relative. 'Organ harvesting', on the other hand, is not a term that is universally known; it is the medical professional's slang for organ donation (for a discussion of the use of this term, see Richardson 1996). These 'insider' categories were sociologically categorized, to avoid falling into straight ethnographic description (Jorgensen 1989). Further, the additional use of concepts derived from a body of social scientific theory allowed the data to undergo a form of abstraction and generalization while remaining essentially humanistic. For example, I made use of the concept of 'social death', described by Mulkay and Ernst in 1991 and by Glaser and Strauss back in 1964. This term was not used by my participants. The inclusion of these theoretical concepts, identified in the data but not actually used by the subjects themselves, confers on the analysis a theory-building status. We can begin to make interpretations, drawing out the culturally specific metaphors of the group under study (Hockey 1990) as well as those of our own academic community. Hockey describes this process as a tacking back and forth between our own world view and that of our respondents.

As a further sophistication, Text-base Alpha also allows us to key-in demographic and other variables. So I was able to tag each interview with variables such as age, sex, profession, etc. The software could therefore be asked to 'decontextualize' – pull-out – coded text from specific people, such as all quotes made by nurses about 'euthanasia' (one of my codes). Similarly, I could obtain statements made by both female and male professionals about what was perceived as suitable 'conduct' (the codename) for newly bereaved next of kin; I was thus able to make gender comparisons in these representations of seemly behaviour. Again, we can see how this software did the donkey work, not the thinking. It was up to me to make meaningful selections of quotations for comparisons and analysis.

Analysing the interviews

The analysis of the in-depth interviews with the bereaved women was undertaken in the same way. Just as I started the analysis of the participant observation by mapping out the social organization of death, with the widows I started my thinking process by writing summaries of the events surrounding the death. To make these precise I needed to read and listen to the long transcripts again. As I did this, I also made memos and developed my coding frame. Here are a couple of examples of the descriptive interview summaries. In line with Attig (1996) I have not only given the women false names but I have also changed certain aspects of their stories to protect their identities.

Kate was 62 years old. She was a housewife. Her husband, a lawyer, had died 11 months before while on holiday. They had been married for 30 years. He drowned while sailing. She witnessed his death and the attempts by her fellow crewmates to save him. Her daughter flew out to help her, but she said that the real help and support came from a local funeral director who was kind and supportive. Although she was not prepared for his death, she felt sure it was a good one. She arranged the funeral. Her daughters and son clearly made every effort to help their mother, but Kate felt very lonely. She had not received any counselling or therapy. She belonged to the Church of England but clearly felt very distant from it. Kate talked intimately and freely. The interview lasted for about three hours.

Christine was about 35 years old. She was unemployed and appeared to suffer from drug or alcohol dependency. Her husband had also been unemployed. He had died eight months previously after ten years of marriage. Keith died of lung cancer. He died, at home, in Christine's presence. She did not feel prepared for his death. She called his death a bad one. The local authority arranged a free funeral for her. Christine was not on speaking terms with her mother or her brother. She had had a child some years before, although I was not clear who currently looked after her son; I guessed he was in care. As far as I could tell she had not received any social support, apart from a couple of visits from her social worker. She had not received any counselling. Christine was disillusioned with the Church. Understandably cynical about my research, Christine was still helpful. She was very upset. As she was also still in pain from a recent operation to her leg, I kept the interview short. It lasted about an hour.

During this time I became vicariously immersed in the world of bereavement and the experience of arranging a funeral. I could have been in danger of becoming locked into the perspective of the bereaved women I was supposed to be 'studying'. So at this stage I returned to the field or looked at the data analysis of the participant observation to remind myself of my perspective as a social scientist.

I developed a different coding frame for the in-depth interviews. The topics covered in these interviews were somewhat different from those touched on by the deathwork professionals, although there was some overlap. The coding frame for the analysis of the widows' text was based on several core concepts, such as the representation of the good or bad death (see Chapter 6). I also focused on the following: cause of death, bureaucracy, spiritual and ritual aspects, the women's social life, her satisfaction with funeral arrangements and various other codes, such as 'advice' (what advice she would give a widowed woman), 'pollution' (statements that suggest she experienced pollution fears concerning the corpse), etc. I used a code for the interview situation, mostly to indicate periods of distress. In both coding frames I had one code called 'bucket' in which I would code interesting statements that did not fit any of the other codes provided. Once again, the code titles, of which there were 48 in total, were based on a mixture of the respondent's own categories and labels, such as 'widow's role' or 'afterlife' and those based on my theoretical or abstract constructs, such as 'pollution', or 'euphemism' (avoidance of topics, or use of euphemism, by participants).

Throughout this book I present quotations from my subjects. The coded text, whether in position in the original transcript or 'decontextualized' by the software package into some list under a code name, provided me with hundreds of natural quotations. I have made an effort to use representative statements, trying to avoid the merely shocking, funny or bizarre. The use of quotations can be problematic. The researcher becomes very familiar with the data and may, at times, use quotations that make great sense to them, familiar with the context in which they were gathered, but to no one else. Despite this risk, however, it is particularly enlightening to let the respondents speak in their own words. People were naturally eloquent when talking about their experiences. Giving my respondents a voice also reminds the reader that my data were based on real lives.

Bibliography

Abric, J. C. (1984) 'A theoretical and experimental approach to the study of social representations in a situation of interaction', in R. M. Farr and S. Moscovici (eds) *Social Representations*, 166–83, Cambridge: Cambridge University Press.

Adams, S. (1993) 'A gendered history of the social management of death and dying in Foleshill, Coventry, during the inter-war years', in D. Clark (ed.) *The Sociology of Death*, 149–68, Oxford: Blackwell.

Agar, M. (1980) *The Professional Stranger*, New York: Academic.

Albery, N., Elliot, G. and Elliot, J. (eds) (1993) *The Natural Death Handbook*, London: Virgin.

Allport, F. H. (1924) *Social Psychology*, Boston: Houghton-Mifflin.

Allport, G.W. (1954) 'The historical background of modern social psychology', in G. Lindzey (ed.) *Handbook of Social Psychology*, vol. 1, 3–56, Reading, MA: Addison-Wesley.

Amir, Y. and Sharon, I. (1982) 'Factors in the adjustment of war widows in Israel', in C. D. Spielberger, I. G. Sarason and N. A. Milgram (eds) *Stress and Anxiety*, vol. 8, Washington DC: Hemisphere.

Ariès, P. (1974) *Western Attitudes Towards Death from the Middle Ages to the Present*, Baltimore: Johns Hopkins University Press.

—— (1983) *The Hour of our Death*, trans. H. Weaver, Harmondsworth: Penguin Books.

Armstrong, D. (1983) *Political Anatomy of the Body*, Cambridge: Cambridge University Press.

Attig, T. (1996) *How We Grieve: Relearning the World*, Oxford: Oxford University Press.

Averill, J. (1982) *Anger and Aggression*, New York: Springer Verlag.

Bachofen, J. (1967) *Myth, Religion and Mother Right*, trans. E. Mannheim, London: Routledge & Kegan Paul.

Ball, J. F. (1977) 'Widow's grief: the impact of age and mode of death', *Omega* 7: 307–33.

Ball, S. J., Bignold, S. and Cribb, A. (1996) 'Death and the disease: inside the culture of childhood cancer', in G. Howarth and P. Jupp (eds)

Contemporary Issues in the Sociology of Death, Dying and Disposal, 151–64, London: Macmillan.

Bauman, Z. (1992a) *Mortality, Immortality and Other Life Strategies*, Oxford: Polity Press.

—— (1992b) *Intimations of Postmodernity*, London: Routledge.

Becker, H. (1958) 'The problems of inference and proof in participant observation', *American Sociological Review*, 23: 652–60.

Becker, E. (1973) *The Denial of Death*, New York: Free Press.

Becker, H. and Geer, B. (1969) 'Participant observation and interviewing: a comparison', in G. J. McCall and J. L. Simmons (eds) *Issues in Participant Observation: A Text and Reader*, 322–31, Reading, MA: Addison-Wesley.

Beier, L. M. (1989) 'The good death in seventeenth century Great Britain', in R. Houlbrooke (ed.) *Death, Ritual and Bereavement*, 43–61, London: Routledge.

Benoliel, J. Q. and Degner, L. F. (1995) 'Institutional dying: a convergence of cultural values, technology, and social organisation', in H. Wass and R. A. Neimeyer (eds) *Dying: Facing the Facts*, 117–39, Washington, DC: Taylor & Francis.

Berger, P. and Luckmann, T. (1967) *The Social Construction of Reality: a Treatise in the Sociology of Knowledge*, Harmondsworth: Penguin Books.

Billig, M. (1986) *Arguing and Thinking: A Rhetorical Approach to Social Psychology*, Cambridge: Cambridge University Press.

—— (1992) *Talking of the Royal Family*, London: Routledge.

Blauner, R. (1966) 'Death and social structure', *Psychiatry* 29 Nov., 379–94.

Bloch, M. (1971) *Placing the Dead. Tombs, Ancestral Villages and Kinship Organisation in Madagascar*, London and New York: Seminar Press.

—— (1982) 'Death, women and power', in M. Bloch and J. Parry (eds) *Death and the Regeneration of Life*, 211–30, Cambridge: Cambridge University Press.

Bloch, M. and Parry, J. (1982) *Death and the Regeneration of Life*, Cambridge: Cambridge University Press.

Bornstein, P., Clayton, P., Halikas, J., Maurice, W. and Robins, E. (1973) 'The depression of widowhood after thirteen months', *British Journal of Psychiatry* 122: 561–6.

Boston, S. and Trezise, R. (1987) *Merely Mortal: Coping with Dying, Death and Bereavement*, London: Methuen, in association with Channel Four Television.

Bowlby, J. (1961) 'Processes of mourning', *International Journal of Psychoanalysis* 42: 317–40.

—— (1971) 'Attachment and loss', vol. 1: *Attachment*, Harmondsworth: Pelican Books.

—— (1975) 'Attachment and loss', vol. 2: *Loss*, Harmondsworth: Penguin Books.

—— (1981) 'Attachment and loss', vol. 3: *Loss: Sadness and Depression*, Harmondsworth: Penguin Books.

Bowling, A. and Cartwright, A. (1982) *Life After Death*, London: Tavistock.

Bradbury, M. A. (1993a) 'Contemporary representations of "good" and "bad" death', in D. Dickenson and M. Johnson (eds) *Death, Dying and Bereavement*, 68–71, London: Sage.

—— (1993b) 'Disposing and remembering: widows' views of cemeteries and crematoria', paper at the Joint Conference of Burial and Cremation Authorities, 52nd joint conference, published in the *Report*, Institute of Burial and Cremation Administration.

—— (1996) 'Representations of "good" and "bad" death among death-workers and the bereaved', in G. Howarth and P. Jupp (eds) *Contemporary Issues in the Sociology of Death, Dying and Disposal*, 84–95, London: Macmillan.

—— (forthcoming) 'Forget me not: memorialisation in cemeteries and crematoria', in *Grief, Mourning and Death Ritual*, Buckingham: Open University Press.

Bronfen, E. (1992) *Over Her Dead Body: Death, Femininity and the Aesthetic*, Manchester: Manchester University Press.

Brown, A. (1987) 'Defining death', *Journal of Applied Philosophy* 4: 155–64.

Burgess, R. G. (1984) *In the Field*, London: Sage.

—— (ed.) (1985) *Applied Qualitative Research*, Aldershot: Gower.

Cain, A. (1972) 'The legacy of suicide: observation on the pathogenic impact of suicide upon marital partner', *Psychiatry* 29: 406–12.

Campbell, D. T. (1969) 'The informant in quantitative research', in G. J. McCall and J. L. Simmons (eds) *Issues in Participant Observation: A Text and Reader*, 289–94, Reading, MA: Addison-Wesley.

Cannadine, D. (1981) 'War and death, grief and mourning in modern Britain', in J. Whaley (ed.) *Mirrors of Mortality: Studies in the Social History of Death*, 187–242, London: Europa.

Cannell, C. and Kahn, R. (1968) 'Interviewing', in G. Lindzey and E. Aronson (eds) *The Handbook of Social Psychology*, 2, 526–95, Reading, MA: Addison-Wesley.

Caplan, P. (ed.) (1987) *The Cultural Construction of Sexuality*, London: Tavistock Publications.

Carey, R. (1977) 'The widowed: a year later', *Journal of Counselling Psychology* 24: 125–31.

—— (1979) 'Weathering widowhood: problems and adjustment of the widowed during the first year', *Omega* 10: 163–74.

Charmaz, K. (1980) *The Social Reality of Death: Death in Contemporary America*, Reading, MA: Addison-Wesley.

Chombart de Lauwe, M. (1984) 'Changes in the representation of the child in the course of social transmission', in R. M. Farr and S. Moscovici (eds) *Social Representations*, 185–209, Cambridge: Cambridge University Press.

Clark, D. (1993) *The Future for Palliative Care*, Buckingham: Open University Press.

Clayton, P. (1979) 'The sequelae and non-sequelae of conjugal bereavement', *Psychiatry* 136: 1530–4.

Clayton, P., Desmarais, L. and Winokur, G. (1968) 'A study of normal bereavement', *American Journal of Psychiatry* 125: 168–78.

Clayton, P., Halikas, J., Maurice, W. and Robins, E. (1973) 'Anticipatory grief and widowhood', *British Journal of Psychiatry* 122: 47–51.

Cleiren, M. P. H. D. (1991) *Adaptation after Bereavement*, Leiden: DSWO Press.

Codol, J. P. (1984) 'On the system of representations in an artifical social situation', in R. M. Farr and S. Moscovici (eds) *Social Representations*, 239–53, Cambridge: Cambridge University Press.

Curl, J. S. (1972) *The Victorian Celebration of Death*, London: Constable.

Danforth, L. (1982) *The Death Rituals of Rural Greece*, Princeton, NJ: Princeton University Press.

Davies, C. (1996) 'Dirt, death, decay and dissolution: American denial and British avoidance', in G. Howarth and P. Jupp (eds) *Contemporary Issues in the Sociology of Death, Dying and Disposal*, 60–71, London: Macmillan.

Davies, D. J. (1996) The social facts of death', in G. Howarth and P. Jupp (eds) *Contemporary Issues in the Sociology of Death, Dying and Disposal*, 17–29, London: Macmillan.

—— (1997) *Death, Ritual and Belief: The Rhetoric of Funerary Rites*, London: Cassell.

Davies, J. (1996) 'Vile bodies and mass media chantries', in G. Howarth and P. Jupp (eds) *Contemporary Issues in the Sociology of Death, Dying and Disposal*, 47–59, London: Macmillan.

Dean, J. P. and Whyte, W. F. (1969) 'How do you know if the informant is telling the truth?', in G. J. McCall and J. L. Simmons (eds) *Issues in Participant Observation: a Text and Reader*, Reading, MA: Addison-Wesley.

Deutscher, I. (1984) 'Choosing ancestors: some consequences of the selection from intellectual traditions', in R. M. Farr and S. Moscovici (eds) *Social Representations*, 71–100, Cambridge: Cambridge University Press.

Dixon, D. (1989) 'Two faces of bereavement: children's magazines and their treatment of death in the nineteenth century', in R. Houlbrooke (ed.) *Death, Ritual and Bereavement*, 136–50, London: Routledge.

Douglas, J. (1985) *Creative Interviewing*, London: Sage.

Douglas, M. (1966) *Purity and Danger: an Analysis of Concepts of Pollution and Taboo*, London: Routledge & Kegan Paul.

—— (1973) *Natural Symbols: Explorations in Cosmology*, London: Barrie & Jenkins.

Duckworth, D. H. (1986) 'Psychological problems arising from disaster work', *Stress Medicine* 2: 315–23.

Durkheim, E. (1898) 'Représentations individuelles et représentations collectives', *Revue de Metaphysique et de Morale* 6: 273–302.

—— (1915) *The Elementary Forms of the Religious Life: a Study in Religious Sociology*, trans. J. Ward Swain, London: Allen & Unwin.

—— (1952) *Suicide. A Study in Sociology*, trans. J. A. Spaulding and G. Simpson, London: Routledge & Kegan Paul.

Elias, N. (1985) *The Loneliness of Dying*, Oxford: Blackwell.

Engel, G. I. (1961) 'Is grief a disease?', *Psychosomatic Medicine* 23(1): 18–22.

Fairbairn, W. D. (1952) *An Object-relations Theory of the Personality*, New York: Basic Books.

Farr, R. M. (1982) 'Interviewing: the social psychology of the inter-view', in F. Fransella (ed.) *Psychology for Occupational Therapists*, 151–70, London: Macmillan.

—— (1983) 'Wilhelm Wundt (1832–1920) and the origins of psychology as an experimental and social science', *British Journal of Social Psychology* 22(4): 289–301.

—— (1987) 'Social representations: a French tradition of research', *Journal for the Theory of Social Behaviour* 17(4): 343–69.

—— (1993) 'Theory and method in the study of social representations', in G. M. Breakwell, and D. V. Canter (eds) *Empirical Approaches to Social Representations*, 15–38, Oxford: Clarendon Press.

—— (1996) *The Roots of Modern Social Psychology (1872–1954)*, Oxford: Blackwell.

—— (1998) 'From collective to social representations: aller et retour', *Culture and Psychology* 4(3): 275–96.

Faschingbauer, T., Devaul, R. and Zisook, S. (1977) 'Development of the Texas Inventory of Grief', *American Journal of Psychiatry* 134: 696–8.

Festinger, L., Riecken, H. and Schachter, S. (1956) *When Prophecy Fails*, Minneapolis: University of Minnesota Press.

Field, D. (1989) *Nursing the Dying*, London: Routledge/Tavistock.

—— (1996) 'Terminal care education for doctors', in G. Howarth and P. Jupp (eds) *Contemporary Issues in the Sociology of Death, Dying and Disposal*, 111–23, London: Macmillan.

Field, D. and Johnson, I. (1993) 'Volunteers in the British hospice movement', in D. Clark (ed.) *The Sociology of Death*, Oxford: Blackwell.

Firth, S. (1996) 'The good death: attitudes of British Hindus', in G. Howarth and P. Jupp (eds) *Contemporary Issues in the Sociology of Death, Dying and Disposal*, 96–110, London: Macmillan.

Flament, C. (1984) 'From the bias of structural balance to the representation of the group', in R. M. Farr and S. Moscovici (eds) *Social Representations*, 269–85, Cambridge: Cambridge University Press.

Foltyn, J. L. (1996) 'Dead beauty; the preservation, memorialisation and destruction of beauty in death', in G. Howarth and P. Jupp (eds) *Contemporary Issues in the Sociology of Death, Dying and Disposal*, 72–83, London: Macmillan.

Foucault, M. (1970) *The Order of Things*, trans. A. Sheridan, London: Tavistock.

—— (1972) *The Archaeology of Knowledge*, trans. A. Sheridan, London: Tavistock.

Foucault, M. (1973) *The Birth of the Clinic*, trans. A. Sheridan, London: Tavistock.

—— (1979) *The History of Sexuality*, vol. 1, trans. R. Hurley, London: Allen Lane.

Frazer, J. G. (1980) *The Golden Bough*, London: Macmillan.

Freud, S. (1957) 'Mourning and melancholia', in J. Strachey (ed.) *Standard Edition of the Complete Psychological works of Sigmund Freud*, vol. 14, London: Hogarth Press.

Fulton, R. (1965) 'The sacred and the secular', in R. Fulton (eds) *Death and Identity*, 89–105, New York: Wiley.

Fulton, R. (1995) 'The contemporary funeral: functional or dysfunctional?', in H. Wass and R. A. Neimeyer (eds) *Dying: Facing the Facts*, 185–209, Washington, DC: Taylor and Francis.

Gardner, K. (1998), 'Death, burial and bereavement amongst Bengali Muslims in Tower Hamlets, East London', *Journal of Ethnic and Migration Studies* 24(3): 507–21.

Geer, B. (1969) 'First days in the field: a chronicle of research in progress', in G. J. McCall and J. L. Simmons (eds) *Issues in Participant Observation: a Text and Reader*, 144–62, Reading, MA: Addison-Wesley.

Giddens, A. (1978) *Durkheim*, London: Fontana Paperbacks.

—— (1991) *Modernity and Self-Identity*, Cambridge: Polity Press.

Gittings, C. (1984) *Death, Burial and the Individual in Early Modern England*, London: Croom Helm.

Glaser, B. and Strauss, A. (1964) 'The social loss of dying patients', *American Journal of Nursing* 64: 119–21.

—— (1965) *Awareness of Dying*, Chicago: Aldine.

—— (1968) *A Time for Dying*, Chicago: Aldine.

Glick, I., Weiss, R. and Parkes, C. (1974) *The First Year of Bereavement*, New York: Wiley.

Glover, J. (1990) *Causing Death and Saving Lives*, Harmondsworth: Penguin Books.

Goffman, E. (1959) *The Presentation of Self in Everyday Life*, Harmondsworth: Penguin Books.

—— (1961) *Asylums: Essays on the Social Situation of Mental Patients and Other Inmates*, Harmondsworth: Penguin Books.

Gold, R. L. (1969) 'Roles in sociological field observations', in G. J. McCall and J. L. Simmons (eds) *Issues in Participant Observation: a Text and Reader*, 30–38, Reading, MA: Addison-Wesley.

Gore, P. (1992) *From Undertaker to Funeral Director: the Development of Funeral Firms in East Kent*, unpublished M.Phil thesis, University of Kent.

Gorer, G. (1955) 'The pornography of death', *Encounter* 5: 49–53.

Hallam, E., Hockey, J. and Howarth, G. (forthcoming) *Beyond the Body: Death and Social Identity*.

Harré, R. (1984) 'Some reflections on the concept of "social representations"', *Social Research* 51: 927–38.

Harris, O. (1982) 'The dead and the devils among the Bolivian Laymi', in M. Bloch and J. Parry (eds) *Death and the Regeneration of Life*, Cambridge: Cambridge University Press.

Heidegger, M. (1962) *Being and Time*, trans. J. Macquarrie and J. Robinson, New York: Harper & Row.

Heider, F. (1958) *The Psychology of Inter-personal Relations*, New York: Wiley.

Hertz, R. (1960 [1905–6]) *Death and the Right Hand. A Contribution to the Study of the Collective Representation of Death*, trans. R. and C. Needham, London: Cohen & West.

Herzlich, C. (1973) *Health and Illness: a Social Psychological Analysis*, London: Academic Press.

Hewstone, M. (1985) 'On common-sense and social representations: a reply to Potter and Litton', *British Journal of Social Psychology* 24: 94–6.

Hochschild, A. R. (1979) 'Emotion work, feeling rules and social structure', *American Journal of Sociology* 85: 551–75.

Hockey, J. (1990) *Experiences of Death: an Anthropological Account*, 129–48, Edinburgh: Edinburgh University Press.

—— (1993) 'The acceptable face of human grieving? The clergy's role in managing emotional expression during funerals', in D. Clark (ed.) *The Sociology of Death*, 129–48, Oxford: Blackwell.

—— (1996) 'The view from the west: reading the anthropology of non-western death ritual', in G. Howarth and P. Jupp (eds) *Contemporary Issues in the Sociology of Death, Dying and Disposal*, 3–16, London: Macmillan.

Houlbrooke, R. (ed.) (1989) *Death, Ritual and Bereavement*, London: Routledge.

Howarth, G. (1993) 'Investigating deathwork: a personal account', in D. Clark (ed.) *The Sociology of Death*, Oxford: Blackwell.

—— (1996) *Last Rites: the Work of the Modern Funeral Director*, Amityville, New York: Baywood.

Humphreys, L. (1970) *Tearoom Trade: Impersonal Sex in Public Places*, London: Duckworth.

Huntington, R. and Metcalf, P. (1979) *Celebrations of Death: the Anthropology of Mortuary Ritual*, Cambridge: Cambridge University Press.

Illich, I. (1976) *Limits to Medicine: Medical Nemesis: the Expropriation of Health*, London: Penguin Books.

Jahoda, G. (1988) 'Critical notes and reflections on "social representations"', *European Journal of Social Psychology* 18: 195–209.

Jalland, P. (1989) 'Death, grief and mourning in the upper class family', in R. Houlbrooke (ed.) *Death, Ritual and Bereavement*, 171–87, London: Routledge.

James, N. and Field, D. (1992) 'The routinization of hospice: bureaucracy and charisma', *Social Science and Medicine* 34: 1363–75.

Jodelet, D. (1991) *Madness and Social Representations*, Brighton: Harvester-Wheatsheaf.

Joffe, H. (1999) *Risk and 'The Other'*, Cambridge: Cambridge University Press.

Johnson, J. (1976) *Doing Field Research*, New York: Free Press.

Johnson, S. (1987) *After a Child Dies: Counselling Bereaved Families*, New York: Springer.

Jorgensen, D. (1989) *Participant Observation*, London: Sage.

Jupp, P. (1993) 'Cremation or burial? Contemporary choice in city and village', in D. Clark (ed.) *The Sociology of Death*, 169–97, Oxford: Blackwell.

Katz, J. T. S. (1993) 'Caring for dying people' in Workbook Three of K260, *Death and Dying*, Milton Keynes: Open University.

—— (1996) 'Nurses' perceptions of stress when working with dying patients on a cancer ward', in G. Howarth and P. Jupp (eds) *Contemporary Issues in the Sociology of Death, Dying and Disposal*, 124–36, London: Macmillan.

Kellehear, A. (1990) *Dying of Cancer: the Final Year of Life*, Reading: Harwood Academic Publishers.

Kelly, G. A. (1955) *The Psychology of Personal Constructs*, vol. 1, New York: Norton.

Klass, D. (1995) 'Spiritual aspects of the resolution of grief', in H. Wass and R. A. Neimeyer (eds) *Dying: Facing the Facts*, 243–68, Washington, DC: Taylor & Francis.

Kubler-Ross, E. (1970) *On Death and Dying*, London: Tavistock.

—— (1975) *Death. The Final Stage of Growth*, Englewood Cliffs, NJ: Prentice-Hall.

Lattanzi-Licht, M. and Connor, S. (1995) 'Care of the dying: the hospice approach', in H. Wass and R. A. Neimeyer (eds) *Dying: Facing the Facts*, 143–61, Washington, DC: Taylor & Francis.

Laungani, P. and Morgan, J. D. (eds) (1998) *Variations in Funerals across Religions and Countries*, London: Routledge.

Laurence, A. (1989) 'Godly death: individual responses to death in seventeenth-century Britain', in R. Houlbrooke (ed.) *Death, Ritual and Bereavement*, 62–76, London: Routledge.

Leach, E. R. (1961) *Rethinking Anthropology*, London: Athlone Press.

Leaney, J. (1989) 'Ashes to ashes: cremation and the celebration of death in nineteenth-century Great Britain', in R. Houlbrooke (ed.) *Death, Ritual and Bereavement*, 118–35, London: Routledge.

Leboyer, F. (1975) *Birth Without Violence*, New York: Knopf.

Lewis, C. (1961) *A Grief Observed*, London: Faber and Faber.

Lindemann, E. (1944) 'Symptomatology and management of acute grief', *American Journal of Psychiatry* 101: 141–8.

Lindzey, G. (ed.) (1954) *Handbook of Social Psychology*, 2 vols, Reading, MA: Addison-Wesley.

Lindzey, G. and Aronson, E. (eds) (1968) *The Handbook of Social Psychology*, 5 vols, 2nd edn, Reading, MA: Addison-Wesley.

Lindzey, G. and Aronson, E. (eds) (1985) *The Handbook of Social Psychology*, 2 vols, 3rd edn, New York: Random House.

Littlewood, J. (1992) *Aspects of Grief: Bereavement in Adult Life*, London: Routledge.

—— (1993) 'The denial of death and rites of passage in contemporary societies', in D. Clark (ed.) *The Sociology of Death*, 69–86, Oxford: Blackwell.

Lofland, J. (1971) *Analysing Social Settings*, Belmont, CA: Wadsworth.

Lopata, H. Z. (1973a) 'Living through widowhood', *Psychology Today* 7: 87–92.

—— (1973b) *Widowhood in an American City*, Morristown, NJ: General Learning Press.

—— (1979) *Woman As Widows: Support Systems*, New York: Elsevier.

Lukes, S. (1973) *Emile Durkheim: His Life and Work*, Harmondsworth: Penguin Books.

Lundin, T. (1984a) 'Morbidity following sudden and unexpected bereavement', *British Journal of Psychiatry* 144: 84–8.

—— (1984b) 'Long-term outcome of bereavement', *British Journal of Psychiatry* 145: 424–8.

McCall, G. J. and Simmons, J. L. (eds) (1969) *Issues in Participant Observation: a Text and Reader*, 322–31, Reading, MA: Addison-Wesley.

Maddison, D. C. and Walker, W. L. (1967) 'Factors affecting the outcome of conjugal bereavement', *British Journal of Psychiatry* 113: 1057–67.

Maddison, D. C. and Viola, A. (1968) 'The health of widows in the year following bereavement', *Journal of Psychosomatic Research* 12: 297–306.

Malinowski, B. (1922) *Argonauts of the Western Pacific*, London: Routledge & Kegan Paul.

Marková, I. (1982) *Paradigms, Thought and Language*, Chichester: Wiley.

—— (1987) *Human Awareness*, London: Hutchinson Education.

Marris, P. (1958) *Widows and their Families*, London: Routledge & Kegan Paul.

—— (1986) *Loss and Change*, Routledge & Kegan Paul.

Mead, G. (1934) *Mind, Self and Society: from the Standpoint of a Social Behaviourist*, C. W. Morris (ed.), Chicago: Chicago University Press.

Mellor, P. A. (1993) 'Death in high modernity: the contemporary presence and absence of death', in D. Clark (ed.) *The Sociology of Death*, 11–30, Oxford: Blackwell.

Middleton, J. (1982) 'Lugbara death', in M. Bloch and J. Parry (eds) *Death and the Regeneration of Life*, 134–54, Cambridge: Cambridge University Press.

Mitchell, M. (1994) 'Lay perceptions of post-traumatic stress disorder', paper presented at the Northern Ireland British Psychological Society conference.

—— (1996) 'Police coping with death: assumptions and rhetoric', in G. Howarth and P. Jupp (eds) *Contemporary Issues in the Sociology of Death, Dying and Disposal*, 137–48, London: Macmillan.

Mitford, J. (1963) *The American Way of Death*, New York: Simon and Schuster.

Morely, J. (1971) *Death, Heaven and the Victorians*, London: Studio Vista.

Morgan, J. D. (1995), 'Living our dying and our grieving: historical and cultural attitudes', in H. Wass and R. A. Neimeyer (eds) *Dying: Facing the Facts*, 25–45, Washington, DC: Taylor & Francis.

Moscovici, S. (1973) Preface to C. Herzlich, *Health and Illness: a Social Psychological Analysis*, London: Academic Press.

—— (1976) *La Psychanalyse: son Image et son Public*, 2nd edn, Paris: Presses Universitaires de France.

—— (1984a) 'The phenomenon of social representations', in R. M. Farr and S. Moscovici (eds) *Social Representations*, 3–69, Cambridge: Cambridge University Press.

—— (1984b) 'The myth of the lonely paradigm', *Social Research* 51: 939–67.

—— (1985) 'Comment on Potter and Litton', *British Journal of Social Psychology* 24: 91–2.

—— (1993) *The Invention of Society. Psychological Explanations for Social Phenomena*, trans. W. D. Halls, Cambridge: Polity Press.

Mulkay, M. (1993) 'Social death in Britain', in D. Clark (ed.) *The Sociology of Death*, 31–49, Oxford: Blackwell.

Mulkay, M. and Ernst, J. (1991) 'The changing profile of social death', *European Journal of Sociology* 32: 172–96.

Nuland, S. B. (1994) *How We Die*, London: Chatto and Windus.

Oakley, A. (1993) *Essays on Women, Medicine and Health*, Edinburgh: Edinburgh University Press.

Orne, M. (1952) 'On the social psychology of the psychological experiment, with particular reference to demand characteristics and their implications', *American Psychologist* 17: 776–83.

Pappas, D. M. (1996) 'Euthanasia and assisted suicide; are doctors' duties when following patients' orders a bitter pill to swallow?', in G. Howarth and P. Jupp (eds) *Contemporary Issues in the Sociology of Death, Dying and Disposal*, 165–78, London: Macmillan.

Parkes, C. M. (1964a) 'Recent bereavement as a cause of mental illness', *British Journal of Psychiatry* 110: 198–204.

—— (1964b) 'The effects of bereavement on physical and mental health: a study of the medical records of widows', *British Medical Journal* 2: 274–9.

—— (1965) 'Bereavement and mental illness', *British Medical Journal* 38: 1–26.

—— (1970) 'The first year of bereavement: a longitudinal study of the reactions of London widows to the death of their husbands', *Psychiatry* 38: 444–67.

—— (1975) 'Determinants of outcome following bereavement', *Omega* 6(4): 303–23.

—— (1986) *Bereavement: Studies of Grief in Adult Life*, Harmondsworth: Penguin Books.

Parkes, C. M. and Weiss, R. S. (1983) *Recovery from Bereavement*, New York: Basic Books.

Parkes, C. M., Benjamin, B. and Fitzgerald, R. (1969) 'Broken heart: a statistical study of increased mortality among widowers', *British Medical Journal* 1: 740–3.

Pollock, G. H. (1970) 'Anniversary reactions, trauma and mourning', *Psychoanalytic Quarterly* 39: 347–71.

Porter, R. (1989) 'Death and the doctors', in R. Houlbrooke (ed.) *Death, Ritual and Bereavement,* 77–94, London: Routledge.

—— (1994) *London: A Social History,* Harmondsworth: Penguin Books.

Potter, J. and Litton, I. (1985) 'Some problems underlying the theory of social representations', *British Journal of Social Psychology* 24: 81–90.

Prior, J. (1989) *The Social Organisation of Death: Medical Discourse and Social Practice in Belfast,* Basingstoke: Macmillan.

Purkhardt, S. C. (1991) 'Social representations and social psychology: a theoretical critique with reference to the psychology of groups 1960s–1980s', 2 vols, unpublished PhD thesis, University of London.

—— (1993) *Transforming Social Representations: a Social Psychology of Common Sense and Science,* London: Routledge.

Radley, A. (ed.) (1993) *Words of Illness: Biographical and Cultural Perspectives on Health and Disease,* London: Routledge.

—— (1994) *Making Sense of Illness: Social Psychology of Health and Disease,* London: Sage.

Ramsay, R. (1977) 'Behavioural approaches to bereavement', *Behavioural Research Therapy* 15: 131–5.

Rando, T. A. (1995) 'Grief and mourning; accommodating to loss', in H. Wass and R. A. Neimeyer (eds) *Dying: Facing the Facts,* 211–41, Washington, DC: Taylor & Francis.

Raphael, B. (1984) *The Anatomy of Bereavement: a Handbook for the Caring Professions,* London: Unwin Hyman.

Rees, W. (1971) 'The hallucinations of widowhood', *British Medical Journal* 4: 37–41.

Richardson, R. (1988) *Death, Dissection and the Destitute,* London: Routledge & Kegan Paul.

—— (1989) 'Why was death so big in Victorian Britain?', in R. Houlbrooke (ed.) *Death, Ritual and Bereavement,* 105–17, London: Routledge.

—— (1995) 'Donors' attitudes towards body donation for dissection', *The Lancet* 346: 277–9.

—— (1996) 'Fearful symmetry: corpses for anatomy, organs for transplantation', in S. J. Younger, R. C. Fox and L. J. O'Connell (eds) *Organ Transplantation: Meanings and Realities,* Wisconsin: University of Wisconsin Press.

Robbins, M. (1996) 'The donation of organs for transplantation: the donor families', in G. Howarth and P. Jupp (eds) *Contemporary Issues in the Sociology of Death, Dying and Disposal,* 179–92, London: Macmillan.

Rose, G. (1982) *Deciphering Sociological Research,* Basingstoke: Macmillan.

Rosenthal, R. (1966) *Experimenter Effects in Behavioural Research*, New York: Appleton.

Rudinger, E. (ed.) (1986) *What To Do When Someone Dies*, London: Consumers' Association.

Samerel, N. (1995) 'The dying process', in H. Wass and R. A. Neimeyer (eds) *Dying: Facing the Facts*, 89–116, Washington, DC: Taylor & Francis.

Sanders, C. (1980) 'A comparison of adult bereavement in the death of a spouse, child, and parent', *Omega* 10: 303–22.

—— (1981) 'Comparison of younger and older spouses in bereavement outcome', *Omega* 11: 217–32.

—— (1983) 'Effects of sudden versus chronic illness death on bereavement outcome', *Omega* 13: 227–41.

—— (1989) *Grief: the Mourning After. Dealing with Adult Bereavement*, London: Wiley.

Scheible Wolf, S. (1995) 'Legal perspectives on planning for death', in H. Wass and R. A. Neimeyer (eds) *Dying: Facing the Facts*, 163–84, Washington, DC: Taylor & Francis.

Schou, K. C. (1993) 'Awareness contexts and the construction of dying in the cancer treatment setting: "micro" and "macro" levels in narrative analysis', in D. Clark (eds) *The Sociology of Death*, 238–63, London: Macmillan.

Semin, G. (1985) 'The "phenomenon of social representations": a comment on Potter and Litton', *British Journal of Social Psychology* 24: 92–3.

Seymour-Smith, C. (1986) *Macmillan Dictionary of Anthropology*, London: Macmillan.

Showalter, E. (1987) *The Female Malady: Women, Madness and English Culture 1830–1980*, London: Virago.

Small, N. (1993) 'Dying in a public place' in D. Clark (ed.) *The Sociology of Death*, Oxford: Blackwell.

Stillion, J. M. (1995) 'Death in the lives of adults: responding to the tolling of the bell', in H. Wass and R. A. Neimeyer (eds) *Dying: Facing the Facts*, 303–22, Washington, DC: Taylor & Francis.

Strathern, A. (1982) 'Witchcraft, greed, cannibalism and death: some related themes from the New Guinea Highlands', in M. Bloch and J. Parry (eds) *Death and the Regeneration of Life*, 111–33, Cambridge: Cambridge University Press.

Strauss, A. (1987) *Qualitative Analysis for Social Scientists*, Cambridge: Cambridge University Press.

Strauss, B. and Howe, R. (1991) *Generations: the History of America's Future 1584 to 2069*, New York: William Morrow.

Stroebe, W. and Stroebe, M. (1987) *Bereavement and Health: the Psychological and Physical Consequences of Partner Loss*, Cambridge: Cambridge University Press.

Sudnow, D. (1967) *Passing On: the Social Organisation of Dying*, Englewood Cliffs, NJ: Prentice-Hall.

Van Gennup, A. (1960) *The Rites of Passage*, trans. M. Vizedom and G. Caffee with an introduction by S. Kimball, London: Routledge & Kegan Paul.

Veatch, R. M. (1995) 'The definition of death: problems for public policy', in H. Wass and R. A. Neimeyer (eds) *Dying: Facing the Facts*, 405–32, Washington, DC: Taylor & Francis.

Volkan, V. (1970) 'Typical findings in pathological grief', *Psychiatric Quarterly* 44: 231–50.

Walter, T. (1994) *The Revival of Death*, London: Routledge.

—— (1996) 'Facing death without tradition', in D. Clark (ed.) *The Sociology of Death*, Oxford: Blackwell.

Wax, R. (1952) 'Reciprocity as a field technique', *Human Organisation* 11: 34–7.

Weisman, A. (1978) 'An appropriate death' in R. Fulton, E. Markusen, G. Owen, and J. L. Scheiber (eds) *Death and Dying: Challenge and Change*, 193–4, Reading, MA: Addison-Wesley.

Wilcox, S. and Sutton, M. (1985) *Understanding Death and Dying*, Palo Alto, CA: Mayfield.

Williams, R. (1990) *A Protestant Legacy: Attitudes towards Death and Illness Among Older Aberdonans*, Oxford: Clarendon Press.

Worden, W. (1991) *Grief Counselling and Grief Therapy: a Handbook for the Mental Health Practitioner*, 2nd edn, New York: Springer.

Wundt, W. (1900–20) *Völkerpsychologie: Eine Untersurchung der Entwicklungsgesetze von Sprach, Mythus und Sitte*, 10 vols, Leipzig: Engelmann.

Yamamoto, J., Okonogi, K., Jurasaiki, T. and Yoshimura, S. (1969) 'Mourning in Japan', *American Journal of Psychiatry* 126: 1660–5.

Zelditch, M. (1969) 'Some methodological problems of field studies', in G. J. McCall and J. L. Simmons (eds) *Issues in Participant Observation: a Text and Reader*, 5–18, Reading Mass.: Addison-Wesley.

Zisook, S., Devaul, R. and Click, M. (1982) 'Measuring symptoms of grief and bereavement', *American Journal of Psychiatry* 139: 1590–2.

Zucker, A. (1995) 'Rights and the dying', in H. Wass and R. A. Neimeyer (eds) *Dying: Facing the Facts*, 385–403, Washington, DC: Taylor & Francis.

Index

T - #0162 - 071024 - C0 - 216/138/14 - PB - 9780415150224 - Gloss Lamination